D1742551

Depression

Anxiety Relief Guide to Comprehend the
Autonomic Nervous System, Learn to Reduce
Stress, Ptsd, Trauma, Autism and Panic Attacks

(Use Polyvagal Theory for Happiness)

Joshua Boyes

Published by Kevin Dennis

© Joshua Boyes

All Rights Reserved

Depression: Anxiety Relief Guide to Comprehend the Autonomic Nervous System, Learn to Reduce Stress, Ptsd, Trauma, Autism and Panic Attacks (Use Polyvagal Theory for Happiness)

ISBN 978-1-989920-83-1

Legal & Disclaimer

The information contained in this book is not designed to replace or take the place of any form of medicine or professional medical advice. The information in this book has been provided for educational and entertainment purposes only.

The information contained in this book has been compiled from sources deemed reliable, and it is accurate to the best of the Author's knowledge; however, the Author cannot guarantee its accuracy and validity and cannot be held liable for any errors or omissions. Changes are periodically made to this book. You must consult your doctor or get professional medical advice before using any of the

TABLE OF CONTENTS

Introduction

Anxiety panic attack is a poignant frame of mind, combining feelings of worry and unpleasant thoughts that give rise to bodily changes, incorporating tension and stress, rise in heart beat rate and changes in blood flow.

People often confuse anxiety disorder with a mental illness. In fact, anxiety is more of a behavioral condition than a mental state. Anxiety attack can take two forms; either be a short term illness or a prolonged trait. Moreover, there is yet another confusion made often between anxiety and fear. Fear is correlated to the precise behaviors of getaway and evasion, while anxiety is the result of threats that are professed to be unmanageable or inescapable.

Anxiety disorder is linked to a condition of excessive anxiety and panic. This is where the patients may experience a sense of dread and panic as well as a feeling of being on the verge of death.

Anxiety and panic pivots on fear and negative assessment and people often debate whether the attacks are related to a kind of social phobia. Anxiety disorder does not necessitate any therapeutic, healing or mental involvement. This is the reason why psychoanalysis and healing treatments have failed to providing any complete resolution to an anxiety panic situation.

When an anxiety or panic attack becomes frequent to the point of enduring beyond the time frame of a stressful condition, one can assume that he or she is facing from an anxiety disorder. In more serious conditions, when the anxiety starts to interfere with nearly all aspects of a daily life, it becomes a disabling anxiety disorder.

This is where people start to make use of excessive alcohol and drugs for short term relief. Addiction to drugs becomes a possibility and the condition of the patient becomes more than just anxiety and panic to deal with.

As we all know, anxiety panic disorder is a mental state, and any treatment aimed at resolving a anxiety attack should first be concentrated towards treating the mental or physical state of the patient.

If you want your anxiety attack problems to disappear forever and you also desire a one time, permanent solution to all your panic attack worries, then this BOOK is meant for you. Everything you think you know about anxiety, worry and panic attack and steps to develop a confident you are fully discussed.

What are you waiting for?

Let's get started!

Chapter 1: What Is Tapping?

EFT and tapping

Emotional freedom therapy (EFT) is a new psychological treatment method, which is widely practiced by people all over the world. Research done on EFT bring to light the fact that EFT is a very effective and efficient method that can help people in multiple ways – it helps treat psychological issues like stress, anxiety and overcome addictions like smoking, drinking, gambling etc. It is also useful for improving your own self-esteem and self-confidence.

This method is based on tapping our meridian points and makes use of scripts to overcome and treat problems. You may use this powerful healing technology either by taking support from a therapist or by carrying out the techniques by yourself. EFT is a type of energy therapy and works in a similar way to other energy therapies like acupuncture, acupressure, shiatsu etc. EFT works by rebalancing energy flow that is as it moves across channels in your body known as meridians.

Research has proven that EFT taps into a section of the brain that stores and processes data, which is used in neurophysiology. Negative thoughts linger as blockages in your brain, which could result in an array of symptoms like fear, anger, stress etc. Some of the causes behind such negative emotions include psychological or emotional disturbances, emotional incidents etc. If you feel that you are inadequately trained, the trauma is too intense, or there is lack of progress, then it would be better for you to get in touch with a qualified practitioner who could help solve your issues and also offer advice on how to improve your own self-practice. I will guide you as best I can in this book but sometimes getting that real life demonstration is much more impactful for learning.

Origins of tapping

Emotional freedom therapy (EFT) has its roots based on therapies like Neuro-Linguistic Programming (NLP), Behavioral Kinesiology and Thought Field Therapy (TFT). There is an interesting story about the origin of TFT, which in turn paved the way for Emotional freedom therapy (EFT).

Dr. Roger Callahan was a cognitive psychologist and hypnotherapist who specialized in phobias. He was researching about Chinese meridians and their effect when you tap at certain meridian points. A patient, Mary, who was suffering from intense phobia of water, came to see Dr. Roger Callahan. He had already tried certain conventional therapies to cure her but was not successful. She complained that she often feels pain in her stomach even when she just thinks about water and her phobia.

Dr. Roger Callahan asked her to tap beneath her eyes for couple of times (this location corresponds to stomach meridian). By applying this seemingly simple technique Mary was relieved of the phobia thanks to the good doc.

Later, Gary Craig who worked with Dr. Roger Callahan in Thought Field Therapy (TFT) started to apply this technique to his patients. He improved some techniques and simplified the process and this adapted method became Emotional freedom therapy (EFT).

In the next chapter we will go into more detail about other treatments and therapies and how they compare to EFT so you can decide which is best for you.

Chapter 2: Face Your Fears

A lady was shopping in one busy street when she suddenly felt uncomfortable. She grabbed for the nearest chair and sat down for a while. This was her first time experiencing this and so she thought that it could just be precipitated by the heat of the sun or the noise around her. When she went to eat in a local restaurant that is full of people, she felt the same thing. She was sweating hard, panting as if she was running out of air and palpitating as if she had just had a strenuous exercise. This happened for another three times in different places. She decided not to go out of the house anymore. Whenever her friends ask her out, she wouldn't join them. Pretty soon, her friends stopped calling her.

The lady was suffering from agoraphobia, a form of anxiety wherein the person does not feel comfortable in crowds. She thinks that a crowded or open place is dangerous. These feelings may or may not be accompanied by panic. This anxiety could be caused by trauma or the presence of stressful factors in one's life.

Many people are being haunted by different fears or phobias – there are fears of open spaces, which the lady in the story has; fear of closed spaces, which is called claustrophobia; fear of heights called acrophobia; or stage fright, which could be manifested as the fear of talking in public. But whatever their fears are, these fears produce the same effect on people. They limit a person's ability to perform optimally.

People with agoraphobia don't get to enjoy playing in theme parks, strolling in the malls, and going to the beach. Claustrophobic people, on the other hand, don't get to work in the office, find comfort at home, and stay in their bedroom. Acrophobic people don't get to enjoy breath taking views from the rooftop of a hotel, don't get to climb mountains and don't get to ride a ferris wheel. Each type of fear stops you from doing what you want and this could affect your life greatly.

When psychiatrists are asked about the best thing to do in cases like this, they give the same answer: you have to desensitize yourself from what you fear most. If you fear open spaces, go out everyday. If you fear talking to a lot of people, join seminars. If you are afraid of heights, go to the top of the tallest building and look at the things around and beneath you. Expose yourself to the sources of your fears. In time, you will cease to be afraid of them and their presence will be normal to you.

Facing one's fears is one of the most difficult things to do. It is like walking in the dark and you don't know what could happen to you. It is like being blindfolded and all you can do is to look for something familiar through your sense of touch. But you don't have to do this on your own.

Sure it is your fear that you have to face, but it doesn't mean that you can't ask for someone's help. If you think that it is too much for you to bear, have someone to support and help you all the way. Don't be afraid to ask for help. There are people around you who are willing to take the journey with you.

Chapter 3: Defining Anxiety

Anxiety is defined as "distress or uneasiness of mind caused by fear of danger or misfortune." There are multiple symptoms as well as types of anxiety and anxiety disorders, but they all have in common is that they all center on the often intense, irrational fear and dread over any given situation, event, condition, feeling or illness. When these symptoms become excessive, you may not just have anxiety, but a specific anxiety disorder.

Anxiety is a very real and very frightening problem. It affects over 40 million adults a year in America alone and, if left untreated, can get much worse. Anxiety is often associated with other mental and physical illnesses and when this is the case, the anxiety may not improve if the underlying illness is not treated first. If you believe you have anxiety disorder, get as much information as you can and seek treatment as soon as possible.

Identifying Anxiety

As mentioned before, there are many types of anxiety and identifying the type(s) that you or someone you love suffers from, is the first step in the treatment process.

Types of Anxiety & Anxiety Disorders:

Generalized Anxiety Disorder

This is the most common anxiety disorder to affect older adults. This anxiety disorder is often a chronic and long-lasting anxiety that has no specific focus. In other words, it often doesn't have a specific trigger, and depression can often be an accompanying condition.

Panic Disorder

Often confused with Generalized Anxiety Disorder, this disorder often shows more of the physical symptoms (sweating, trembling, dizziness, nausea, labored breathing, etc) and is an ongoing and usually sudden occurrence of panic attacks which are usually described as intense terror. The American Psychiatric

Association (APA) defines this disorder as fear or discomfort that abruptly arises and peaks in less than ten minutes. It can last for several hours and can be triggered by stress, fear, or even exercise, and the specific cause is not always apparent to the anxious person.

A diagnosis of this type of anxiety disorder often requires that the panic attacks are ongoing and carry the fear of what each attack will cause: severe dread of future attacks, and how one starts reacting to their attacks. The sufferer may start to show physical symptoms (with no panic attack even occurring) and will often focus on what the attack is causing their body to do therefore believing that their health is in question.

Panic Disorder With Agoraphobia

This condition rears its ugly head when a panic attack or attacks come about in specific geographic locations. It will often cause the sufferer to be a prisoner in their own home.

Phobias

This is the most common form of anxiety and can take the form of a fear of any specific situations or stimuli.

Agoraphobia

Closely-linked with Panic Disorder, this condition leads to one being extremely afraid to leave their home (or other "safe zone") because of a feeling of inability to "escape" any given situation or location. This can be intensified if the sufferer has had a panic attack in the particular setting before.

Social Anxiety Disorder or Social Phobia

This disorder usually manifests itself as a fear of humiliation or embarrassment in social situations. It can be a fear of something specific, such as public speaking, or could be any social situation whatsoever. In its more severe cases, it can lead its sufferers to complete isolation.

Obsessive-Compulsive Disorder

Often referred to as OCD, it can become a life-altering and debilitating condition. It's characterized by a seemingly-inescapable "need" to repeat an act or "ritual" sometimes associated with distress if not completed.

Post-Traumatic Stress Disorder

Also known as PTSD, this anxiety disorder that can come about from a very serious situation such as a trauma in combat, rape, a car accident, a tragic death, etc. PTSD can be accompanied by avoiding people, places, and things, and experiencing flashbacks, anger, depression and more.

Separation Anxiety

Expected to a degree in children and babies, this condition can become excessive when it leads to panic attacks at even brief separations from an individual or location. Adults can experience Separation Anxiety Disorder at the end of a significant relationship.

Some Symptoms of Anxiety:

This is a comprehensive list of some of the most common symptoms:

Irregular or intensified heartbeat

Shortness of breath or hyperventilation

A feeling of disconnect from reality

A perceived feeling of impending death

Tingling in the lips

Tingling in the hands and fingers

Uncontrollable trembling and/or chills

Dizziness

Nausea

Sweating

Weakness

Feeling faint

Chest pains

Becoming flushed

A feeling of loss of control

A perceived feeling of a heart attack

Feeling of "losing your mind"

Some Clinical Treatments for Anxiety

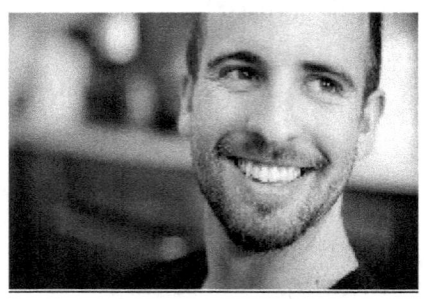

There are many different effective treatments and therapies for anxiety disorders and new treatments are being explored and discovered constantly as research continues.

A specific form of therapy may prove completely useless to one person that is practically a life-saver to another. With the help of physicians, psychiatrists and psychologists/therapists, anxiety can be dealt with effectively. This handbook will teach you ways to cope with your anxiety and do so with many different available methods. It will help you to reduce its impact, lessen its frequency, loosen its hold on you and allow you to function

more normally. You can lead a fulfilling
life.

Chapter 4: The Many Faces Of Fear

In essence, fear is an illusion inexistent in the physical world; but it exists in our minds and manifests through our actions. There are certain fears that the great majority of human beings share.

Let us look at the top 5 countdowns of certain human fears that every member of a society deals with throughout their life.

Failure

Though failure is a very ambiguous and subjective term and its meaning varies from person to person depending on one's perspective, the fear of failure deserves the top spot because it rules over all our actions and decisions. We all do or don't do things in order to avoid failure. The main fear of failing comes with the disappointment that follows, that feeling that despite your effort, nothing seemed to go as you wished it did, and it causes feelings such as "why bother?" or "I'm just not good enough".

That is why this is the worst fear of all, the fear or failure is very often used as an excuse to procrastinate, or not do anything to make situations better.

Fear of Loss-Things/Freedom/Death

We often hold on to our owned things because we are afraid to get rid of them. We're afraid to give up what we think we have.

No one wants to feel that absence of **things**, and this has caused the media to feed us more of this fear through advertisements, telling us that we need more things than we actually do .We don't just fear the loss of these things that we think we might rather we fear the loss of what these things might potentially mean to us in some distant hypothetical future. That puts us in misery – the extreme case of poverty where we are unable to cover our own basic personal needs due to the lack of resources. Misery is considered as the lowest point in what comes to human needs, and that is why we fear it so much.

Though the human mind doesn't think about the fear of losing **freedom** every single moment, there are times when the mind wonders as to what would happen if we were to lose the power to control our own lives. Childhood memories of being grounded in your room by yourself without the possibility of leaving until you finished your homework or our fear of the commitment in relationships and marriages are classic examples.

The **fear of one's own death** is tightly tied to the fear of the unknown; we can just speculate about what happens to us when we leave this world but we are never sure about it. This fear does not make it to the topmost position, because it is a well-known truth that we all in the end will kick the bucket. We avoid the thought of it as a near future occurrence in our lives and hence, subconsciously we do not consider death as our worst everyday worry.

Fear of Social Acceptance- Ridicule, Rejection and Loneliness

The fear of social acceptance is similar to the fear of loss except for the fact that it is not about losing stuff than one possesses; rather it is about losing one's social existence. So we fear loss of acceptance, loss of friends, loss of love and similar other losses pertaining to societal behaviours.

One of our early survival instincts makes us think that it is more likely that we would survive if we live in-group. Most of us can only justify our existence through the acknowledgement and acceptance of others.

We fear that not behaving "correctly" and in accordance with the cultural norms will result in our rejection from the 'social' group.

Also, the fear of not projecting a good enough image of ourselves to others causes the fear of ridicule- the fear of getting bad criticism in any form of mockery such as laughter or, in the worst cases, booing. We all have experienced this form of fear at least once in our lives, often through a common experience called the "stage fright", when we have to speak or perform in front of an audience.

The fear of being alone is that dreadful feeling of emptiness caused by the absence of interaction with other human beings. We tend to judge the meaningfulness of our actions based on the attention that they get from other people around. We end up thinking –"So what if I made a groundbreaking discovery, no one else has acknowledge or appraised it, does it still count?"

Such 'social fears' prevents us from becoming trendsetters. But again, we do not like the feeling of being in the spotlight for a negative reason, and being at the mercy of the opinions of others. As a result we tend to (sometimes blindly) follow the actions of others and go with flow rather than challenging their meaning and relevance in our lives.

The Unknown

The human mind fears losing control over one's life and its situations. Our mind tells us that in order to move forward, we must know what is waiting for us there, because only then can we control and establish a measurement that we can use to manipulate the result of our actions.

This paves the path for the fear of the unknown. We do not like what is different because beyond our understanding and beyond control.

A classic example that most of us can relate to is that as kids we are afraid of the dark, mainly because we did not know what might be hiding in the darkness.

This fear poses a hindrance for us in terms of our discovering and understanding new things; it encourages the need to pull ourselves away from it and hence, induces closed mindedness.

Pain

The physical pain can be described as an unpleasant sensation, generally caused by damage to a certain body part. Though the intensity of physical pain is a purely subjective feeling, and it varies from person to person individual, in general, most of us are intolerant or afraid of physical pain.

It is a well-known fact that there exists great amount of medications related to pain relief, related to different types of pain.

The fear of pain gives rise to the fear of losing one's freedom owing to the physical immobility that a person might face when a particular part of the body is injured. We tend to keep away from certain actions that cause us pain as it is one of the key elements in survival instinct, and also because our brain tells us that the actions we are doing is causing a negative effect on our bodies.

Pain may be a dreaded and an undesired feeling but it is not a bad thing in itself; it lets us know what we must stop doing that we are doing to avoid further damage to our body.

Chapter 5: Fundamental Relaxation Techniques

It would be wise for you to find the time to learn to relax. You will be doing your body and mind a big favor. After all, stress can demand so much of your thoughts and time such that it has led you to believe that relaxing will make you less productive. This cannot be farther from the truth, for relaxation is a necessary part of life. It lets you recharge, clear your thoughts, and make way for more meaningful thoughts instead of your constant worries.

Write it All Down

The first step to relax is to find out how stressed you are. Becoming more knowledgeable of your current condition lets you take a step back and assess things objectively. This step alone will already make you feel more in control of the situation. Once you have gauged your stress levels, you can now identify the causes. You can keep a journal where you can list down the causes and record your daily experiences with stress. Does your anxiety have to do with your relationships, your health, finances, social life, work, or worry about the future? You can efficiently manage these sources by pinpointing them in your journal and letting you take action more efficaciously. Choose a small notebook which you can carry around with you, or you can download an app to keep a record of it.

Writing it all down does not mean that you have to relive the moment; you simply need to make a note of the situation. Right after you have jotted it down, rate its importance to your life on a scale of 1 to 10, with 10 as being extremely important. Oftentimes, the 8 to 10s have to do with major financial losses, the death of loved ones, dangerous illnesses, and so on. The 4 to 7s would be situations such as your car breaking down or losing cash. The 1 to 3s would be getting stuck on traffic, having to deal with a rude salesperson, or forgetting your umbrella at home when it's about to rain.

Naturally, you would not want to take note of every single stressor in your life. You only write in your journal when you feel the need to do so, and not necessarily after you have just experienced the stressful situation. However, you must avoid making excuses from taking the time to objectively assess your stress levels. Pick a time of the day, usually right before you go to bed, to write down your thoughts in your stress journal if you feel that you will be too busy.

Take Deeper Breaths

The simplest way for you to calm yourself down is to apply the right breathing techniques. Controlling your breathing will allow your body to take in a healthy amount of oxygen and flush out the carbon dioxide from your blood. Your diaphragm is the one that is responsible for your breathing and while it is on autopilot, it does not cooperate very well when you are feeling stressed and your breathing becomes shallow and fast. You will need to turn to manual during these times.

To test your current way of breathing, lie down on your back and place your hand over your stomach. Breathe like you normally do and check to see the rise and fall of the hand on your stomach. The more significant it is, the better you are at natural breathing. If your breaths are short, then you will need to become more conscious of how you breathe. You can also practice this basic breathing technique: sit or lie down comfortably, place one hand on your abdomen and the other on your chest. Breathe in through the nose, allowing the abdomen to rise but not the chest. Slowly exhale through slightly parted lips at a count to four, letting your abdomen fall gradually. The trick is to practice Abdominal Breathing for this allows your body to take in the maximum amount of oxygen that it can handle and to exhale as much carbon dioxide as possible.

When you are under pressure, there is another breathing relaxation technique that you can do as well. You can call this 911 Breathing. To do it, you first breathe in through your nostrils and fill up your lungs and your cheeks, making them puff out. Hold this in while mentally counting from 1 to 6 seconds. Then you release it all out through your mouth in the shape of a small "o". After that, you pause for a little bit and then breathe like you normally do. You can repeat doing this exercise until you feel relaxed, which usually takes place on the third repetition.

Stretch and Relax your Body

Once you have learned how to breathe more effectively, you can now move on to a relaxation technique that will release the tension from your muscles. This is called Deep-muscle Relaxation and it is a technique that conditions your body to adapt to tension.

To practice this, you will be tensing a particular muscle group in your body, such as your back, your shoulders, limbs, and so on. It is such a simple trick but the results are immediately gratifying.

Find a cool and quiet place to do this exercise. Sit or lie down comfortably and close your eyes. Begin with one arm, tighten your hand into a fist, and then stretch it out and tense your muscles for 10 seconds. Keep it tensed as you bend and flex your arm within those 10 seconds. Be careful not to put too much strain on it though. After 10 seconds immediately release the tension and allow your arm to go limp. Observe how your arm will feel after this exercise. Notice how relaxed it is now? Revel in this period for half a minute. Then, you can repeat this exercise to all of the other muscle groups, one at a time.

You can also apply this technique to your facial muscles. Start by scrunching up your forehead and letting your ears pull themselves backwards for about 5 seconds before you let them go. After that, you can stretch out your mouth into a clenched teeth grin for 5 seconds and then relax. Follow it up by puckering up your lips to an extreme "duck face" for 5 seconds and then release.

To do this exercise on your neck and shoulders, begin by pressing your chin down toward your chest and hold that for a few seconds. Then, bend your head to the side on one side and then the other, feeling the tension on your neck. Finally, tilt your head back in a slow and controlled manner and hold it for a few seconds before you release.

Chapter 6: Effects Of Narcissistic Abuse

The residual effects of any abuse can be devastating, however, when most people think about abuse - be it spousal, parental, etc. - they tend to focus on physical abuse. Mental and emotional abuse can be just as if not more damaging, especially when the abuser is someone close to the abused.

Perhaps the worst type of abuse comes from the hands of those who are so preoccupied with themselves that they fail to see or care about the results of their actions.

This type of narcissistic abuse can be found in many different types of relationships including parent-child, spouse/significant other, and even friendships.

Emotional abuse by a narcissistic parent can be especially insidious as it may damage the child's ability to form stable relationships in the future.

It has been proposed that due to a lack of an appropriate model of a healthy relationship, those who suffered emotional abuse as children tend to end up in similar abusive relationships as adults.

Most of the individuals we think of when we think of this period in time were not true narcissists in the strictest sense. The term narcissism is derived from the Greek story of a Naissus, a hunter who was the son of the river god Cephissus and the nymph Liriope.

He possessed such beauty that even he himself could not be free of the attraction. The god Nemesis tricked him into gazing into a pool whereupon he saw and fell in love with his own reflection, only to die there contemplating his own fair features.

Narcissists believe that they can do no wrong, so any problems with the relationship - and even problems which arise in day to day living - are the fault of the other partner. If a mistake is made, the partner is somehow the one to blame.

The narcissists' need for attention and admiration lead them to constantly seek out those who will reinforce their inflated sense of self-worth. This translates to a series of short relationships and a long stream of discarded partners.

If the narcissist is married, there is a high probability that he or she will not be faithful. Naturally, if infidelity is discovered, the partner will be to blame for not being pretty enough, caring enough, etc.

Victims of a narcissistic abuser often display similar characteristics. The most common is a poor sense of self-worth, often accompanied by an inability to make decisions for themselves. They spend years of being told that they are not good enough, not smart enough, not something enough.

Over time they come to internalize these negative statements. They doubt their own abilities. This makes them more reliant upon the narcissistic abuser, creating a cycle of co-dependency.

This is one of the most troubling aspects of narcissistic abuse in terms of parental care. When children are constantly belittled, they grow up believing that they are not capable.

When they are finally out from beneath the control of their narcissistic parent, they lack the coping skills required to survive on their own.

Doubting their own decision making abilities and crippled by poor self-esteem, they gravitate towards someone who will accept them despite their self-perceived flaws and make decisions for them.

In short, they enter into relationships with narcissistic abusers. They leave their parents only to end up with someone exactly like the very people who abused them in the first place.

Those who have suffered at the hands of a narcissist may display any number of emotional and physical symptoms which may be difficult to attribute to the relationship as they are a result of the stress they face daily. These include confusion, disassociation, poor eating and sleeping habits, and even signs of Post Traumatic Stress Disorder (PTSD).

It is especially difficult for those in a relationship with a narcissist to get help as they have become conditioned to looking to their abuser for most if not all decision making activities. Their poor sense of self worth makes it easy for them to ignore the idea that they deserve better.

Obviously, in their minds, no one else would have them. They should be happy with the relationship they have, despite the fact that they are unhappy. This is a theme which the abuser will reinforce as well.

While difficult, it is possible to escape the cycle of narcissistic abuse. The first step must be accepting that no one deserves the constant humiliation and demands of the narcissist. As the self-image is restored to a healthy level, it becomes easier to make decisions without the abuser's input. Naturally, this is an extremely difficult process which may require the help of outsiders including professionals. Unfortunately, it is common for narcissistic abusers to restrict their partners' access to others, especially those who would express opinions which run contrary to their grandiose sense of self.

Chapter 7: Where Does Your Social Anxiety Come From?

Before looking for solutions to your social anxiety, it's a good idea to examine the source of the problem. And, actually, knowing where your social anxiety comes from can help you deal with it more effectively. This chapter guides you as you consider the reasons you might have trouble in social situations.

Genetics

Some people are just naturally more social than others. According to Arlin Cuncic, an expert on social anxiety, about 30% to 40% of the root cause of social anxiety is genetically based. If someone in your immediate family has social anxiety disorder, you are 30% more likely to have it than someone who doesn't.

Brain Chemistry

People with social anxiety usually have different levels of certain brain chemicals than those who don't. These brain chemicals, called neurotransmitters, include serotonin, norepinephrine, dopamine, and gamma-aminobutyric (GABA). Your doctor can do tests or learn through observation the extent of the imbalances of these brain chemicals and prescribe medications to help balance them out so you can feel less social anxiety.

Brain Structure and Blood Flow

Research studies have shown that the blood flow in certain parts of the brain is different for people who have social anxiety than for people who don't have social anxiety disorder. In general, these are the parts of the brain affected by anxiety: the brain stem is in charge of your heart and respiration rates, the limbic system controls your mood and anxiety level, the prefrontal cortex is the part of the brain that makes it possible for you to assess risk and danger levels, the motor cortex controls your muscles.

All of these brain structures influence the way you respond to social situations, and if your doctor were to do a PET scan, it would show increased blood flow in the parts of your brain that are most active. In fact, one study did use the PET scan to see the difference in the brains of people with and without social anxiety disorder as they spoke in public. In the people with social anxiety disorder, the blood flow was dramatically increased to the amygdale, a part of the limbic system excited during fear. The people who didn't have social anxiety had no extra blood flow to the amygdala, but instead, their increased blood flow was to the cerebral cortex, allowing them to focus on thinking and evaluating the situation calmly.

Behavioral Disinhibition

Behavioral dishinibition refers to a pattern of interaction during childhood. It happens when the child is a toddler or slightly older. What happens is that the child displays more emotion than other children, especially when they are in a new situation. These toddlers often grow up to have social anxiety when they are adults. The best possible solution if you see these warning signs in your child is to seek professional help for them.

Family Social Patterns

The way you and your family members interacted with each other during childhood can play a big role in whether you have social anxiety later in life. If one of your parents displays fear in social situations, you might pick up on and mimic that fear, even if you aren't genetically inclined to social anxiety. You see what your parent does and imitate the behavior. And, in fact, it is natural to mimic your parents' behavior when you are very young. This is how you learn. But, if your role models are socially anxious or awkward, their example isn't a helpful one.

Social Trauma

Did you have a very distressing social experience at sometime in your past? Even the most socially-adept person can become socially anxious if they have been through a traumatic social experience. The good news is that, if you weren't socially anxious before the event, you have a very good chance of getting back to your feeling of social ease. In a case like this, it's best to see a professional for therapy sessions to help you deal with the trauma.

Social Anxiety Isn't Who You Are

One thing to remember as you consider why you have social anxiety is that you aren't defined by this condition. It's something that holds you back from expressing the fullness of your true identity. As soon as you start confusing your anxiety condition with your true identity, you stop the process of getting beyond it. After all, if it's who you are, you can't change that. But, it's not really who you are. It's a condition you can change, whether through therapy, medication or learning new techniques to deal with it.

Spend a few moments right now listing your personal qualities, accomplishments and hopes. For this exercise, don't write anywhere on your list anything about your social anxiety. Keep your list so you can refer to it in the future any time you start to think of yourself only as someone with social anxiety.

You might never really know why you have social anxiety, but examining the possible causes can help you understand the problem better. And, it can help you realize that social anxiety doesn't make you less of a person or inferior in any way. It just means that you have to go through a learning process before you can conquer your social fears.

Chapter 8: Opening Yourself To New Possibilities

If you are feeling stuck, frustrated, or unmotivated, you should re-think the way you are living your life. Your social anxiety may be preventing you from opening yourself to new possibilities. Hence, you should change the way you view the world and the people around you. You should consider getting out of your comfort zone in order to experience what the world has to offer. How can you do this?

Get Out of Your Head. Just stop overthinking things. A lot of people become anxious because they keep on overthinking things. They become paranoid and overly concerned of what other people have to say about them.

Let us say that you are in class and the professor calls on you. Unfortunately, you were not able to study the previous day which is why you could not answer the question. The professor starts to embarrass you in front of the whole class, and then the bell rings.

In this situation, do you either get out of the classroom and act as you normally would or do you head straight home and sulk about what just happened. If you do the latter, then you may have a bigger problem in the long run. You see, if you keep on overthinking things, it eventually becomes a habit. Each time something unexpected happens to you, your mind automatically starts to overthink.

You may become paranoid. You may think that your professor and classmates think that you are stupid. You may harbor this false belief that they are talking about you behind your back. You may even think that they are plotting something against you.

Well, having such thoughts is incredibly unhealthy. Not only will it hurt your personal relationships with these people, but you may also put yourself at risk of health problems. When you think too much, you begin to lose sleep and this can lead to a variety of medical conditions.

So, you should just get out of your head and accept the fact that you cannot please everybody. While it may be true that others may talk about you behind your back, you should remind yourself that not everybody does this. Most of them may actually be too pre-occupied by their own issues that they do not even remember your embarrassing experience at all. You should just move on and let bygones be bygones. Overthinking will lead you nowhere.

Challenge Your Beliefs. Always remember that what you believe in can come true. Have you heard of the Law of Attraction? Well, this law states that the more you think of and believe in something, the likelier that it come true. So if you strongly believe in something, you can expect that thing to turn into reality.

If you believe that you can do something no matter how little your success rate may seem, you can certainly accomplish it. Let us say that you really wanted to win a contest but your friends think that your odds of winning are slim. Despite of what they think, you still practiced and performed your best. You also fully believed in yourself. In the end, you won the contest.

You winning the contest is actually a combination of your positive thinking, willpower, and action. Because you believed that you can win, you did your best. You exerted effort and not just imagined yourself getting the trophy.

Then again, you should realize that not everything is possible. There are some things that are just not meant to happen, no matter how hard you wish or hope. For instance, your spouse decided to divorce you. While you can try things that might change her mind, you still cannot manipulate his decision. You can try to woo her with flowers, but you cannot force her to do as you wish.

The same thing goes when you lose a loved one. If your best friend died, there is absolutely nothing you can do to bring him back. No matter how hard you wish or how often you pray, you just cannot bring a dead person back to life.

Nonetheless, there is still something you can do to make yourself feel better. You just have to accept what happened and move on with your life. Your divorce may be devastating, but you still have a future ahead of you. The death of a friend may leave you feeling very hurt, but you are still alive. Do what is best for your life.

Search for Opportunities in Tough Situations. Interacting with other people is tough, and having social anxiety makes this even tougher. Whenever you are faced with a stressful situation, you should avoid playing the victim.

You have to get rid of that poor victim mentality and start to look at the bright side of everything. This will not only help you become more sociable, but it will also help you open yourself up to greater possibilities.

Let us say that your flight has been cancelled. Of course, this gets you agitated. You become frustrated because you have already made your schedule for the week. Not being able to fly to your destination immediately messes up your entire schedule.

Instead of becoming anxious, you should see the bright side of this situation. Why not use your waiting time as a time to relax? You can read a good book, for instance. It can help you learn new things and develop better perspectives in life. If not for your cancelled flight, you may have never had the opportunity to read that book that would change your life forever.

A similar example is when you lose a job. Of course, losing a job is devastating. It puts you in a position in which you do not know how you will put food on the table. Well, while you have not yet gotten a new job, you should use your free time to improve yourself.

You can start working on your skills so you can have a higher chance of getting hired. You can also consider starting a business, create a business plan, and study the market. In addition, you can use this time to hang out with friends and be with your family members. When you were busy with work, you may have neglected your children. Now is the perfect time for you to catch up with what is going on with their lives.

Eliminate the Things That No Longer Work for You. In order to move forward with your life, you should get rid of whatever holds you back so you can make room for something better. You have to learn how to let go.

For instance, if you are stuck in a relationship that is unhappy and unhealthy, you should end it. Do not be afraid of not being able to find something better. That is the whole point of letting go. You have to end things that are no longer good for you and open yourself up to new possibilities. This includes accepting that you can be at risk of failure. You may or may not find someone better. Nonetheless, the important thing is that you have tried. Also, you have made the right decision by sparing yourself the agony and pain of being stuck with a person who does not value your needs. Besides, you should not spend all your energy on another person. You have to love and care for yourself first. If you love yourself, you will not stay with people who hurt you.

Try New Things. People with social anxiety are usually afraid to try new things because they are afraid that other people will judge them. If you have social anxiety, your disorder might have prevented you from enjoying new things and going on adventures your whole life.

As a child, you may have always wanted to dance in a recital. However, your fear of failing and being judged may have prevented you from doing so. Now that you are older, you should not give up on your dream. In order to overcome your social anxiety, you should give yourself a chance to dance.

If you are worried about embarrassing yourself in public, you should practice instead. You can hire a dance instructor to help you out. You can also practice at home when no one is watching. As you become better at dancing, the more confident you become. Confidence is important in battling anxiety. Eventually, you will feel that you are ready to dance in public.

Chapter 9: Tip #2: Before The Exam—

Develop Good Study Habits

The first tip that you need to do is to develop good study habits. Studying hard for the exam is not enough. You also need to study right to be able to retain the information that you have learned while studying. The most important thing is to remember what you have learned while you are taking the exam. You may have studied hard, but it is useless if you do not remember any of the information that you have learned when you are already answering the test. It is important to develop good study habits that will help you perform well during the exam. Here are some good study-habit tips that you need to know.

Set a schedule for studying

Examination schedules are usually announced weeks before the test itself. This gives you plenty of time to prepare. Sadly, some people always procrastinate when the exam date is still weeks away and end up cramming for it (often the night before the examination date). What you can do is set a schedule for studying right after you learn about the date of the examination. If you are a student, you can review your lessons every night just to keep your mind "refreshed". You can plan a major weekly review every weekend, wherein you have to study the topics that your teachers have discussed the past week. If you are an employee who needs to get a test for a certification, you can schedule your review at least an hour or day after work, or every weekend. The most important thing is to stick to your schedule no matter what, and make sure that you only study on your set review schedule.

Avoid distractions

While studying, you should avoid any distraction that will keep you from focusing on the task at hand. Disconnect your laptop from the internet or do not use your laptop at all. Turn off your mobile phone and your TV set to keep your attention focused. You should also avoid eating meals like spaghetti, which is messy and requires your attention when eating. In addition, crackers keep you from hearing your own thoughts because of the loud sound that they produce when you munch on them. If you prefer munching while studying, you can eat something like nuts and grains, or small chocolate candies that you can easily pop into your mouth and will not create too much noise. It is also important to study inside a closed room where people cannot talk to you, so that you can concentrate on studying.

Use memory tricks

Many people use different kinds of memory tricks to remember important information that may be asked when they take the exam. One popular example of a memory trick is the mnemonic device, like ROYGBIV (which stands for the seven colors of the rainbow). This is an effective way to remember lists or groups. You can also use the association technique, wherein you associate two different things to remember an important piece of information – like associating your birthday or your loved ones' birthday with important dates in history. By using these memory tricks, memorizing information becomes a lot easier, helping you a lot when the test comes.

Take down notes

Notes are very important when it comes to studying. Many people use their own notes to study rather than relying solely on their textbook or printed handouts given by the teacher. What's the reason behind that? It's because they find their notes more effective. While listening to your teacher, a lecturer, or a speaker, it is important to write down important notes because these can help you remember things later when you are already studying. Notes also allow you to highlight the things that you need to concentrate on. When studying for an exam, writing down notes is also an effective way to retain information. According to studies, a lot of people remember information better when they write them down instead of simply reading or hearing the information.

Study with a friend

Any activity is more fun if you do it with a friend, and that includes studying. You can ask each other some questions to test your knowledge about the subject matter. Explaining theories with someone is much better in terms of retention than simply memorizing things alone. Studying with someone also allows you to share information and knowledge that you may have missed if you were studying alone. Just make sure that you do not distract each other from studying. Do not gossip or play video games during study time. You can do anything you want once your time for studying is over.

Make studying more fun and interesting

Instead of simply reading your notes and memorizing things, you can make studying more fun and interesting using different techniques. For instance, you can make flashcards with pictures to help you jog your memory about certain topics. You can also draw comics that narrate the story of WWI and WWII. When taking down notes, you can use colorful markers to underscore the important things that you need to remember. Studying need not be boring contrary to popular belief.

Chapter 10: Learning The Art Of Small Talk To Overcome Shyness And Meet People

As indicated in the previous chapters, one of the things shy people do is stay away from any situation that requires them to have an actual interaction with another person. In effect, their shyness creates a wall between them and everybody else. This may seem convenient in the short term, but over the long run, chronic shyness has the potential of turning into a bigger, far worse problem.

In most cases, shyness can be alluded to one's longstanding fears. The fear of getting rejected, the fear of disappointing others, and the fear of humiliating oneself can cause somebody to retreat into a silent and safe corner where they feel they are the least vulnerable from other people's stares. At its most extreme, this tendency to withdraw from social interactions can lead to social phobia -- a crippling fear of interacting with other people.

But just like anything else, the best way to overcome shyness is by facing it head on. The usual and most convenient practice of running away from your fears does nothing to solve the problem at hand. Instead, doing so only serves to validate and perpetuate such fears.

Light and casual talk

In the case of shyness, one of the best ways to overcome it is by subjecting yourself to situations that you would otherwise avoid or find difficult. This need not be a drastic decision. For example, if you find it tough to speak before a crowd, don't start with a huge audience. The key to expanding any comfort zone and developing new skills is to start small with a foundation and build on the foundation piece by piece. Start with small groups and work your way up from there. As you begin to get comfortable in stretching your comfort zone you will grow your social muscles.

Engaging in small talk is one of those things that may seem easy to do, but is in fact more complicated. Small talk is just that -- a supposedly easy, noncommittal, light, and casual conversation between two people who hardly know each other. It can be used to either kill time or mark the beginning of something great, such as an enduring friendship, a business deal, or a possible romantic partnership.

Emphasis should be placed on light and casual. Don't put completely unnecessary pressure on yourself by thinking that this is a test and you will be judged. Otherwise, you're just inviting stress and in the process aggravating your shyness.

Pumping yourself up

Your body reacts accordingly to environmental stimuli. If you are under a stressful situation, such as one where your shyness is triggered, your heart rate becomes faster and you begin to breathe more than usual. If you want to engage in small talk, you must first ensure that your body is doing fine.

Thankfully, there are a couple of basic relaxation techniques that can help you be more at ease. One of these is deep breathing. The main purpose of this exercise is to bring your heart rate to normal levels. You start by breathing in through your nostrils. Hold your breath for five seconds before slowly breathing out through your mouth. Do this repeatedly until you have fully calmed down. If there is space available and you have extra time to spare, you can also try out a number of alternative relaxation practices, such as yoga, meditation, and Tai'Chi.

Other people resort to quick and unconventional strategies to shake off stress. For example, some people lock themselves up in the bathroom and jump up and down or else do some stretching exercises to feel more relaxed. Others scream at the top of their lungs to release all the pent-up tension. Others choose to be more discreet by holding onto and squeezing a stress ball or looking at anything green to feel more relaxed. Many people have a musician or a certain song that can help them alter their state. Experiment with different sources to find what works best for you.

Sporting an 'open stance'

People tend to shy away from people who look unapproachable. A key to initiating a conversation with anyone is by projecting an open stance. This means that your demeanor should be warm and accommodating, not someone who looks irritated or someone who can't be bothered. You should be able to make a good first impression; people normally spend just a couple of seconds to decide if someone is worth talking to. Those few seconds are critical, so you should learn to take full advantage of them.

To sport a confident demeanor, begin with the basics: mind your posture. Avoid slouching. Keep your body straight when you are sitting or walking. Studies show that people who willfully follow proper posture feel more confident than those who don't. Similar studies show that individuals with proper posture are likelier than others to be looked up to, especially since a regal stance is almost always identified with power, wealth, and intelligence.

So if you are someone who struggles with shyness, observing proper posture provides you an extra boost of much-needed confidence.

A big part of having an open stance is sporting a friendly smile. This is a classic sign of confidence. When you smile, you are telling the world that you are doing great, are friendly and open to a new conversation or interaction.

Engaging and interesting

Perhaps the biggest challenge to initiating small talk is what to say to the other person. But instead of struggling over how to get started, try out a couple of safe and direct introductions. For example, "Hi, my name is X. What's your name?" is a quick and standard introduction to get things started unobtrusively. Now that you've got that out of the way, here are a few pointers to keep in mind:

☐ Choose a common topic. The weather is probably the most overrated subject for small talks, but there's a reason why it remains a popular choice: it's never the same and it affects everybody. Other good conversation starters are the quality of the coffee you're drinking or the food you're eating, as well as the city that you were born and raised in. You can also get started by stating a sincere compliment about the other person. Everyone likes compliments and that puts the focus on the other person, not yourself. Just make sure it is genuine.

☐ It's good to be informed of the news or other topics of general interest. There's a good chance the other person is aware of such topics and may even harbor interesting opinions. The key is to just get the conversation going.

☐ Be on the lookout for verbal or visual cues. Be observant. Is there something on his or her shirt that indicates what his or her interests are? What about the books he or she brings? Is there any topic he or she said that you are familiar with or interested in? Take time to look at your surroundings, too.

Ask open-ended questions, or those that require more than a single-worded reply. This way, the other person can expound a bit more and you can pick up hints as to what to talk about. This can be one of your most powerful tools. Most people love to talk about themselves and love it when others listen. As they answer your questions, you will receive more information about the person to keep the conversation going and serve as a basis for additional questions.

It's fine to talk about yourself, but refrain from giving out too much information. It is important that you share a part of yourself as a way of getting the conversation going. However, you need to learn the divide between appropriate and inappropriate. The rule of thumb is: don't open up about something that you would be uncomfortable talking about with your own mom or boss at work.

Sport an interest in what the other person has to say. Simple gestures, such as nodding or raising follow-up questions, are two ways to show that you are actually paying attention to what the other person is saying. Maintaining eye to eye contact is just as crucial in this regard.

Refrain from being offensive. Remember that small talks are meant to be casual and light. Don't ruin the vibe by going overboard and committing the usual pitfalls, such as asking too personal questions, making sexual innuendoes, constantly correcting the other person, and disagreeing far too frequently than is necessary.

Use humor for effect. A good joke is a great way to introduce laughter into the conversation. Shared happiness even over something as trifle or inconsequential as a joke creates a more memorable moment, which could serve as a gateway for something more profound. Even making fun of yourself can be a way to lighten any mood.

Learn how to say goodbye properly. Even though you've just met, it still behooves you to be courteous when leaving. Do not walk or run off in an abrupt fashion without saying goodbye. Say something like, "I'd love to keep talking with you, but I have to leave." If everything is going well and you want to continue that same conversation some other time, you can ask for the other person's contact information. See Chapter 5 to read more about following through.

While engaging in small talk, ensure that you are speaking clearly and audibly. There are a lot of things that you can do to improve your speaking skills. If you are not confident with the way you talk, devote some time to practice. You can talk to yourself in the mirror and pay attention to your mannerisms and facial expressions. You can also record your voice to find out how you sound like. The more aware you are of yourself, the better positioned you are to identify your weak points and implement strategies to correct them. Don't worry if you don't like the way you sound when recorded. Our voices always sound different than in "our own head". Nobody is concerned about the sound of your voice.

Similarly, be mindful of your manners and gestures. Sport a confident demeanor without coming across as either too aggressive or too self-absorbed. Remember that this is not just about you. For example, tinkering with your phone while the other person is talking can come across as disrespectful. Putting your arms across your chest and constantly interrupting the other party is a clear sign of rudeness. Pay close attention to these little things.

Most importantly, remain true to yourself. In more ways than one, making small talks is an exploration of what is possible. Aside from being a good exercise to rise above your shyness, it is also a great opportunity to put yourself out there, make new friends, get on dates, be exposed to different personalities, and lend an appreciation to how far you've gotten to conquer your imagined fears. Donning a fake personality isn't going to cut it.

Chapter 11: Conquering Stress With

Mindfulness

Are you sometimes stressed, worrying about trivial things, anxious about any outcomes, feeling uptight at home or at work, restless, sleepless, or fatigued? Is your mind chattering too much? Do you know how to truly relax and find inner peace?

Stress is an issue that can take a toll on your mental and physical health. Occasional stress can be a good thing, but it is not natural for the mind-body when it is exposed to stress-induced hormones for prolonged periods. The negative reactions associated with long-term exposure to stress are too numerous to mention. Add to that lack of exercise, a poor diet and poor environmental conditions and you have a recipe for illness.

Modern life has a tendency to create stress that leaves us entangled in worry and anxiety as fatigued or paralyzed victims of the mental, emotional and physical stress symptoms. If we are to move out of the downward psychological spirals or self-defeating circles - we need to identify what causes the stress and/or take action to avoid reacting to it. We can learn stress management tools that prevent the mind-body from reacting with madness. It is not enough to simply be told to relax.

Key to De-stress

We need the key to unlocking the thoughts and emotions behind our stress and learn to cope to build more resilience, awareness, and strength in our daily life. There are ways to manage time and reduce stress, simultaneously. Most people will say, this is not entirely possible because they are too busy, and do not have the time to use or learn any stress management techniques. The question is, can we afford not to when our mind-body reacts. You can get the 'de-stress key' with mindfulness.

Mindfulness - mindfulness meditation in particular - works to reduce stress. Scientific studies show that Mindfulness Based Stress Reduction (MBSR) can reduce up to 40 percent of our daily stress with many other health benefits. It relieves anxiety, pain and depression, and can help us become more mindful and aware of how we can appreciate life and learn to live in the moment.

Mindfulness Based Stress Reduction

When mindfulness reduces stress, it alleviates many of our modern lifestyle's breathless symptoms. MBSR works in two ways: It helps your mind and thus body to relax properly. When relaxation kicks in the adrenaline and cortisol levels associated with prolonged stress decrease almost immediately. This, in turn, affects the prefrontal cortex so that we can handle emotional triggers; use our planning skills and time more efficiently than when feeling anxious or stressed. In this way, we can learn to strike a balance between positive stress and ordinary (negative) stress due to too many demands on our life and time.

When experiencing stress, the things that you do automatically, the opposite of a mindful awareness, are called stress reactions. If you are lucky, some of your reactions may be helpful and therefore dissipate the stress. More often than not, though, reactions to stress are unhealthy and lead to further stress.

Your reactions to stress are partly based on what you assimilated in childhood, partly genetic, and partly based on your own experiences with stress. If whoever brought you up reacted in a certain way to stress, you have a greater chance of behaving in a similar way.

Your own experience of ways of dealing with stress also comes into the equation. Perhaps you have always drunk several cups of coffee when you are feeling stressed, and find the caffeine helps you to get your work done. Although you may feel this is effective, caffeine is a stimulant and the more you drink, the more stressed you will become.

Reacting automatically implies a lack of choice. Through practicing mindfulness, you begin to have a greater choice of responses, and can thereby achieve a more satisfactory outcome.

Make a list of the unhelpful and helpful ways you deal with stress:

1. Unhelpful reactions may include drinking too much alcohol or caffeine, negative thinking, zoning out, working even harder, or eating too much or too little food.

2. Helpful responses may include going for a walk, exercising, meeting up with friends, meditating, or listening to music.

3. Become more aware of the choices you make following a stressful event, and begin choosing small, helpful strategies such as going for a walk. Make use of

mindfulness skills to help you to make wiser choices.

Here is the two-step mindfulness process for responding rather than reacting when you feel your stress levels rising:

Notice your current reactions. What are your body, mind and emotions doing? Are they showing the signs of stress? Acknowledge the fact that you are suffering from stress. Observe how you are reacting to the stress. Your body may be tense in certain places. Perhaps you are suffering from indigestion or have had a cold for weeks. Your behavior may be different to usual. You may be snapping with anger for the smallest thing. You may not be making time to meet up with friends. Your emotions may be fluctuating. You may feel tired or out of control. Your thoughts may be predominantly negative. You may have trouble concentrating. At this stage, you need to become aware of what is happening, without judging the situation as bad or wrong—just be aware, without the judgment. By becoming aware of what is happening within you, the experience is already transforming. This is because you are observing the stress, rather than being the stress. As the observer of experience, you are no longer tangled up in the emotions themselves. You cannot be what you observe.

Choose a mindful response. Now, from an awareness of the level of stress you are experiencing, you can make a wise, mindful choice as to the best way to cope. You know yourself better than anyone else – you need to decide how best to cope with the stress. As you become aware of your own inner reactions, you make space for creative action to arise rather than habitual, well-worn paths you have chosen many times before.

Here are ten suggestions for a mindful response to your stress:

1. Exercise - The main objective is to find a physical activity that works for you. For example, a 20-minute jog around your

neighborhood can lift your spirits and mood. Walking in the great outdoors can change your perspective and is one of the best forms of exercise. It is also free.

2. Socialize - Spend time with friends and family. It is all too easy to get caught up in daily life and neglect the people who give you a sense of belonging. Schedule time with family and friends and remember how good it feels just to be you around people you love, unwind and have a good time. Having some fun with them may provide all the stress relief you need.

3. Identify Stressors - Dedicating a period of time every day to write about what is bothering you may give you stress relief. Keeping a journal can help you solve many problems or find positive angles around the stressors.

4. Meditate - Learn to practice meditation. Preferably daily before you feel the tension rising. Meditation eases and dissipates mental worry when you are able to take a moment to center yourself and

ease any negative emotions. The benefits of mindfulness meditation are enormous to your mind, body, and emotions.

5. Self-Care - Find ways to nurture yourself with healthy food and proper sleep. When tension spikes, it can be tempting to put yourself last, but prioritizing "me time" with healthy eating, relaxing activities, relationships and adequate rest - is necessary if you want to avoid making your stress worse.

6. Breathe - If you feel stuck or cannot leave the work-desk, take a few minutes to focus on your breath. Take 5-10 slow, deep, full breaths or step outside. This has an immediate calming effect on your mind and body. Taking the time to breathe properly improves your mood and helps you de-stress and relax.

7. Kindness - When you catch yourself thinking negatively about yourself or others, turn your thinking around. Say to yourself: "He /she cannot help it", or "I am doing the best I can at this moment!" Be

kind or loving! It is too easy toget caught up in daily life and neglect yourself. Treat yourself to a nice cup of tea at the end of the day, an occasional body massage, or a holiday with loved ones.

8. Simplify - Life can be full of too many distractions - like gadgets and objects. If your life is cramped up or overloaded with stuff, try to find ways to get rid of what you do not want or really need. Learn to disengage from entanglements.

9. Thankfulness - Showing that you appreciate people and things for the good and support they bring to your life has a powerful, positive effect. It is impossible to feel negative when you are feeling grateful for the things you currently have in your life. Being thankful gives your life perspective and attracts more of what you are joyful or happy about.

10. Allow Change - Sometimes the best way to relieve stress is to remove your source of tension. If you are working at a pace or in an environment that is difficult

due to your boss, colleagues, and so on to earn more money, you might be better off doing something else.

Chapter 12: The Brain And Danger

The three areas of the brain that play a primary role in processing stressful, survival-related experiences are the brain stem, the hippocampus, and the amygdala. The amygdala is the alarm centre in the limbic system which warns us about danger. When it is strongly aroused it stimulates the hippocampus, another part of the limbic system, which is capable of storing large amounts of survival-related memories, as well as the brain stem, which has a direct influence on how the body reacts to danger. This information often takes the form of "somatic markers." These are subconscious procedural memories for stressful events (such as tensing the stomach when being shouted at, or raising the hands when being physically attacked). As well as storing information related to specific traumatic events, the hippocampus and brain stem also store memories for particular emotional states. For example, terror is often connected with a choking feeling in the throat and cramping in the stomach, while joy is often associated with a feeling of warmth and a release of tension in the chest. In general, negative emotional states are strongly focused around the stomach, chest, and throat because in survival terms, these are the areas that are most crucial to our survival and are vulnerable to injury from predators and rivals.

In humans and other primates, simple body states (such as tension in the shoulders and jaw) can also be interpreted as social emotions. Hence, personal situations that threaten our social status, such as rejection, shame, and negative judgment by other people, can cause us to react in the same way as if we are being physically threatened. This mental trait is controlled by a part of the limbic system called the insula, which allows us to sense social emotions like love, hate, guilt and embarrassment.

Chapter 13: 30 Minute Fat Burning Yoga

"Yoga is about balance, both mind and body, as well as increasing self-awareness, with by-products of better strength and flexibility,"says M.E. Dahkid, the author of"Yoga: The Essential Guide: How to Master Weight Loss, Stress Reduction and Find Inner Peace."

The sequence comprises of a couple of warm-up exercises to oxygenate your body and prepare it for the postures that follow. There are around 13 postures, which you need to practice at least two rounds so as to boost your metabolic rate. The sequence ends with Corpse Pose that would help you summarize the whole practice and reap the benefits.

Warming Up with Breathing & Stretches

Sit down in a comfortable seated position, keeping the spine erect, neck and shoulders relaxed, palms resting on the knees with the tips of index finger and thumb touching each other. Close your eyes.

Inhale and expand your belly. Exhale and pull your navel in and close to your spine.

Feel the air moving in and out of the belly, energizing your core and body for the practice.

Do 5 such rounds.

At the end of 5 rounds, lift your legs off the mat, keeping the knees straight, and allow it to come parallel to the floor.

Extend your hands parallel to your legs. Keep the spine nice and long and ensure that your sit bones are resting on the mat. Engage the abdominal muscles and buttocks firmly.

Inhale and stretch backward and rolling your shoulders back. Keep the neck and face relaxed. Stretch back until you are a couple of inches of the floor and your body resembles a low boat.

Exhale and lift your torso making 45 degree angle with the mat. Your body will resemble a high boat. As you come back to this position, feel the core being pulled in towards the spine.

Do 10 rounds.

As you exhale at the end of the 10th round, place your legs on the mat, keeping the knees bent.

Hug your knees with your hands.

Inhale and stretch back on the mat, holding the knees. Exhale and come back to starting position.

Do 5 such rounds.

At the end of the 5th round, place your palms on either sides of the feet and walk your feet backward. Push your hips to the ceiling and heels to the floor.

Inhale and as you exhale, jump or walk in between the palms, keeping your head down and close to the shin.

Inhale, sweep your arms over your head, and lift your torso to take a subtle backbend.

Exhale and join your palms at heart center.

Separate your feet and keep your hands away from the body. Close your eyes and take 5 deep breaths to prepare yourself for the sequence.

20-Minute Weight Loss Sequence

The sequence starts and ends with Tadasana.

1. Tadasana–Samsthithi or Equilibrium Pose

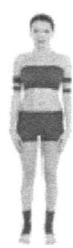

This pose helps to concentrate your thoughts and create an awareness about your body.

How to do:

Stand on the front of the mat, feet touching each other and firmly placed into the mat.

Keep your spine erect, hands joined at your heart center. Keep the neck and head relaxed.

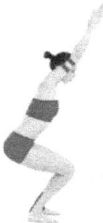

2. Utkatasana—Chair Pose

Tone your legs and sculpt your abs while strengthening your spine and back with this pose.

How to do:

Inhale, and bend your knees until fingertips touch the mat.

Sweep your hands over your head and join your palms.

Push your hips back like you are sitting on a chair and adjust the knees in such a way that it is stacked over the ankles.

Pull your navel in and close to the spine.

Hold the posture for 5 deep breaths.

3. Parivrtta Parsvakonasana - Revolved Side Angle Pose

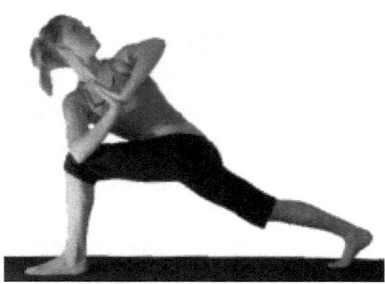

This is a simple twist that works towards improving your digestion. It also tones your torso.

How to do:

Inhale and stretch your right leg backward. Keep the toes tucked.

Exhale, twist to your left, and bring your arms outside of your left knee, keeping the palms joined.

Hold the posture for 5 deep breaths.

4. Anjaneyasana–Lunge Pose

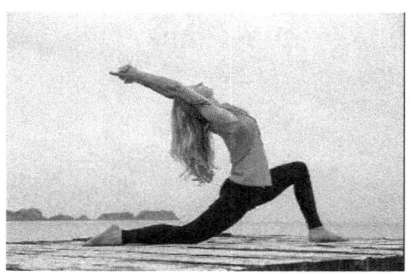

It strengthens and tones your thighs and quadriceps, while toning your abdominal muscles and back.

How to do:

On the final exhalation of Revolved Side Angle Pose, place the right knee down, extending the toes backward.

Inhale and sweep your hands up and over your head, joining your palms. Push the hips squared and down and close to the mat. Keep the left knee stacked over the ankle.

Take a gentle backbend, tilting your head back to gaze at the fingertips. If you have high blood pressure, dizziness or neck issue, keep your head and neck straight, fixing your gaze at a point in front of you.

Hold for 5 deep breaths.

5. Kumbhakasana–Plank Pose

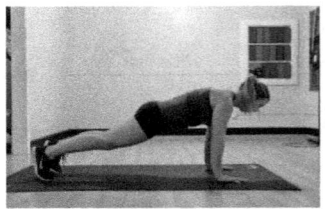

Tone your core, legs, and arms with this wonderful arm balance.

How to do:

With the final exhalation in the Lunge, lift your right knee off the mat, tucking the toes.

Inhale and place your left leg back and close to the right leg, keeping the toes tucked.

Align the wrists in such a way that they are stacked under the shoulders. Spread the fingers wide and strong.

Engage your core, glutes, and quadriceps, and roll back the shoulders.

Gaze forward and hold the posture for 5 deep breaths.

6. _Vasisthasana–Side Plank Pose

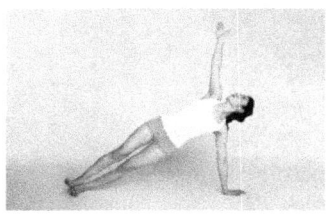

It tones and strengthens your arms, belly, and legs. It is also beneficial to improve your balance and awareness.

How to do:

Inhale and twist to your right, stacking your right feet over the left.

Exhale and lift the right arm up. Hold the pose for 2 deep breaths.

At the end of second exhalation, come back to the Plank pose.

Inhale and twist to your left, stacking your left feet over the right.

Exhale and lift the left arm up. Hold the pose for 2 deep breaths.

At the end of second exhalation, come back to the Plank Pose.

Repeat 5 times on each side.

7. Kumbhakasana

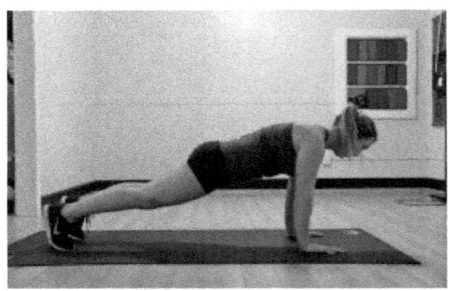

At the end of the final round, come back to the Plank Pose.

8. Bhujangasana–Cobra Pose

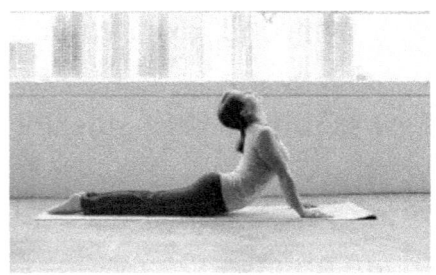

A simple backbend, it heals and strengthens your back muscles.

How to do:

From the Plank, exhale and lie down on the mat on your tummy, keeping the elbows bent and off the floor, yet close to your body. Keep the toes extended backward.

Inhale, push the palms firmly into the mat, and lift your head and torso, till your navel off the mat, and bend backward gently.

Hold the posture, straightening the elbows, and gazing up for 5 deep breaths.

9. Adho Mukha Svanasana–Downward Facing Dog Pose

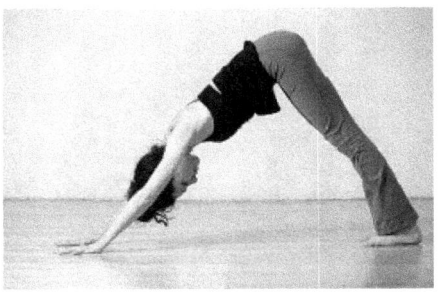

It stretches your arms and legs and promotes relaxation and peace.

How to do:

On the final exhalation in the Cobra pose, tuck your toes and lift your body off the floor.

Push your pelvis and hips towards the ceiling, heels move towards the mat.

Spread the palms wide and stack the wrists under the shoulders, your head coming closer to the mat, in between the elbows.

Hold the posture, engaging the core muscles for 5 deep breaths.

10. Uttanasana–Standing Forward Fold

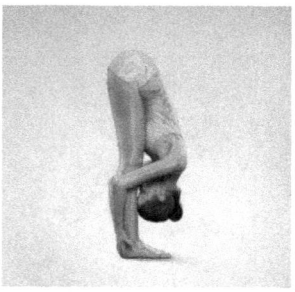

This posture works on your abdomen and helps in improving the flexibility of your hamstrings. A good stress-buster, it helps in toning your back and thighs also.

How to do:

With the final exhalation in Downward facing dog pose, walk or jump in between your palms, and fold forward, allowing your head to come close to the feet.

Keep your knees bent, if you have a bad back or knee injury. Keep the palms wherever they are, either flat or on the fingertips.

Hold the posture for 5 deep breaths.

11. Utkatasana–Chair Pose

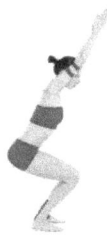

How to do:

Inhale and bend your knees, pushing the hips back like you are sitting on a chair, and stacking the knees over the ankles.

Exhale and sweep your hands over your head, joining the palms.

Hold the posture for 5 deep breaths.

12. Ardha Chakrasana—Half Wheel Pose

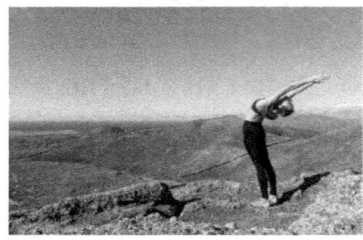

This is a backbend which helps in easing the tension experienced by the body and strengthens your core.

How to do:

Inhale and straighten your knees and torso.

Take a gentle backbend, sweeping your arms over your head, joining the palms.

Hold the posture for 5 deep breaths.

13. Tadasana—Equilibrium Pose

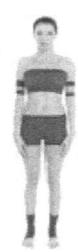

How to do:

Exhale and release your hands on either sides of the body.

Bring your body to a neutral state, keeping the spine erect, head and neck relaxed.

What to do next?

This makes only half of one round of the sequence. Take 5 deep breaths before you move into the other half.

Repeat the sequence once more, changing sides to left in the following postures.

☐ Parivrtta Parsvakonasana

☐ Anjaneyasana

While doing Side Plank, do it on the left side first.

Do the sequence one more time, repeating on either sides for better results, pausing for 5 deep breaths between repetitions.

Wind Up With Savasana

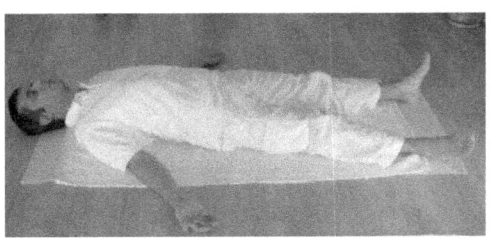

Winding up after a strenuous routine is essential to allow your body and mind to come back to its normal state. Savasana, or Corpse Pose, is a classical restorative pose that allow you to revisit your practice mentally and gather the learning.

How to do:

Lie down on the mat on your back.

Separate your legs wider than your hips, allowing the feet to fall to the sides naturally.

Keep your hands about 12 inches away from the body to allow the armpits to breathe.

Tuck your chin slightly in to give space for your armpits.

Close your eyes and relax, breathing deeply.

Let abdomen rise as you inhale and fall as you exhale.

Revisit your practice mentally, without any judgment, and witness it to gather your learning.

Once you feel you are ready, gently move your toes and fingers. Turn your head from side to side.

Inhale and lift your hands over your head.

Retain the breath and stretch your entire body.

Exhale, roll to your right, and sit down in any comfortable posture, keeping the eyes closed.

Rub your palms to generate heat.

Place your palms on the eyes and slowly open the eyes to the light.

Start practicing this 30 minute session right away and let the excess pounds melt away!

Chapter 14: Herbs

Herbs are known to help with treating anxiety. There are many types of herbs that have been known to help with this illness and have been used and researched for several years. Some herbs help with anxiety right away and others will kick in overtime. So, just be patient and if you feel as if the first herb you try doesn't work, then try a different herb before taking medicine.

Herbs and natural remedies are great for anxiety disorders, because you can not get addicted to these herbs, they are generally free of side effects, and they won't change your personality like medications tend to do.

If you are pregnant or breastfeeding it is not advisable to take any of these herbs, before speaking to a doctor. As there has not been enough research applied to any of these herbs while pregnant or breast feeding, so do not chance taking any of these before talking to a physician. There is not enough evidence of these natural herbal remedies to help children, so make sure to consult with a doctor before giving any of these herbs listed below to anyone under the age of 18.

All of the herbs listed below should not be taken or mixed with other herbs or medications before speaking to a doctor. Also, do not consume any alcohol while taking any of the herbs listed below.

Here are a list of the different types of natural herbs to help relieve anxiety with a list of different ways to take these herbs such as; capsules, teas, and tinctures. Tinctures are made from the plants oils and are very strong. Some of these herbs are powerful or even more powerful than prescription and over the counter drugs for anxiety.

Lemon Balm

Lemon balm has been used for over a thousand years to help with getting rid of anxiety. This herb extracts medicinal ingredients that are known to have a sedative effect calming the human brain and helps with getting the bad thoughts out of your mind which are causing your anxiety. Lemon balm is one of the most popular herbs for helping with anxiety.

The leaves from the lemon balm are used in different types of medicines. Being on edge or feeling nervous can be tiresome. Researchers have found that this herb is extremely helpful when dealing with anxiety, because it calms the nerves.

How to take this herb: Take two leaves from the lemon balm and cut them in half. Pour hot water over the leaves into a mug for hot tea. If you want to make a chilled drink, take one ounce of the lemon balm leaves and mix it with a quart of water. Let it sit for two hours in the refrigerator and then drain. Add some honey to it if you would like. Lemon balm is also sold in a capsule form in health stores. Do not take more than three capsules a day of lemon balm.

Lavender

Lavender has been researched and is known to be just as effective as medicines such as, Valium and lorazepam, but without the side effects of these drugs. Lavender helps with nervousness and restlessness. Not only does lavender help with anxiety it also helps with depression.

How to take this herb: Lavender essential oils come in a liquid form. I personally like to light a candle with the lavender oil above the candle and place a few of these around the house. It makes me feel very relaxed breathing in the lavender scent. Make a warm bath and put about five drops of the lavender oil into the water. Another way to enjoy this herb is by putting it into hot tea by taking whole dried lavender flowers and placing them into boiling water and strain the water before drinking. Lavender capsules are available in health stores and these are called, "Lavela." Taking the capsules may make you feel drowsy, it is better to try making hot tea or placing the oils into a hot bath before trying the capsules.

Valerian

Valerian is an herb, but medicine is made from the root. Valerian is a great herb to help with anxiety. Not only does Valerian help with anxiety, but it is also used as a sleeping aid. Valerian acts like a sedative to the brain and nervous system. This herb is useful for someone who has social anxiety, as it helps to reduce stress in social situations. Valerian root contains complex B-vitamin and magnesium, which also increases calmness to the brain.

How to take this herb: Buy Valerian root capsules in 500mg. Take three of these capsules spread out through the day. Also, making hot tea with Valerian root; boil hot water, pour the water over the dried Valerian root, and steep for about ten minutes. If you are having trouble with sleeping, I suggest drinking a cup of Valerian root hot tea before going to bed.

This tea has always helped me get a good nights rest.

Hops

Hops is a plant and the dried flowers from the plant are used to make medicine. Not only is this herb used to flavor beer, it is also a great source for relieving anxiety. The flowers from the plant are a nerve sedative. Hops is also very helpful if you are having trouble with sleeping at night.

How to take this herb: Taking dried flowers from the hops plant, placing one ounce into a quart of boiling hot water, strain the water, and let it sit for about five minutes. Hops tea has a relaxing and soothing effect on the body. There are capsules of hops and with that, no more than 100mg-200mg should be consumed daily. Also, taking the flowers from the herb and placing them into a pillow case will help calm your anxiety and this is known to help with sleeping.

Passion flower

Passion flower has been researched and it has been found that the chemicals in the herb have a calming effect. Passion flower doesn't show any toxicity. Taking passion flower will not act in a negative way with any other medications. This herb is extraordinary with relieving anxiety and jittery nerves. Passion flower is a wonderful herb to help relax the body.

How to take this herb: In stores you can find passion flower hot tea bags, so drink a cup of this hot tea when anxiety is coming on or when you are feeling stressed. There are capsules of passion flower found in drug or health stores. There are tinctures made up of passion flower. I personally like to put two drops of the passion flower tincture into my orange juice in the mornings. I used to put four drops into my juice, and noticed I was feeling a little more relaxed than what I wanted to, so try two drops at first and if later on you feel as if you would like more, just put one more drop in your juice or you can put it into hot water.

Chapter 15: Say Goodnight To Insomnia

Do you occasionally feel that you have sleep deprivation? Is the quality of your sleep what it needs to be or do you wake up feeling tired and lacking energy? In addition, do you have trouble focusing and just not feeling up to par the rest of the day?

According to the World Health Organization, one third of the world's population experience insomnia at a few point in their life. Of that one third, about five per cent need medical treatment. Beneath are natural techniques and remedies that could help you sleep without the aid of medical intervention.

Before going to bed, take the time to just sit and calm down. Listed to a few soft music, and do many deep breathing exercises. It is additionally greatest to steer clear of caffeine, alcohol, and nicotine.

Developing a bed time routine every

evening will ultimately associate the routine with sleep. For example, you could begin with a cup of hot milk every evening and a warm bath. Milk contains a protein called tryptophan, which assists to promote sleep. A warm bath or shower will lower your internal body temperature again telling your body that it is time for sleep. If hot milk is not for you, try chamomile tea, which is known to calm the nerves.

Watching Television, reading and eating in your bedroom does not promote sleep, thus your body won't associate your bedroom with sleep. Your bedroom ought to be dark and cozy room that makes you feel secure and comfy. The bedroom should make you crave sleep. It is challenging to sleep whenever you mind is full of stuff that you have to do tomorrow. To be able to alleviate this, write a to-do list for the following day. Organize your clothing for the morning and prepare lunches the night before.

Consider making your appointments a bit later in the day in case you have a tendency to worry about getting up in the morning.

Many of us have anxieties and regrets or events from the past that might still haunt us. Issues such as these affect are sleeping patterns. Whatever the issues are, today may be a good time to finally set things straight; forgive that person, forgive your self, give back that item, start speaking with that family member again (or even make that appointment to see a psychologist if necessary).

In addition, you could organize your life and chores, thus making the time for a good nights sleep. For example, make one huge supper and freeze half for an additional day, spot clean the home and pick up daily before it becomes a big job, plan a menu for the week thus alleviating the disappointment of what to cook for supper every night. You owe it to your health and those around you to obtain a good night sleep. With a bit bit of planning and routine, you will get to bed earlier and get the sleep you need. As always, a well-balanced diet makes a well-balanced mind. Whilst you are planning your menus for the week take into account that the meals you are preparing have the important vitamins and minerals. Next, throw away all the junk food, pop and other foods which are loaded with calories but offer no nutritional value. Throw in a bit exercise and your insomnia will progressively fade away with an improved body and mind. If you can't sleep, then get up. Laying in bed worrying that you can't fall asleep will simply make it worse. Get up, go into a different room, and do something to disturb your self until you feel sleepy. Many medications will interfere with your sleep. Check with your medical doctor if you are experiencing insomnia and are additionally taking any of these medications - amphetamines (diet pills), antidepressants, beta blockers (heart and blood tension), cimetidine (ulcers), clonidine (blood tension), cortisone, diuretics (fluid), levodopa (parkinsons), methyldopa (blood tension) and ventolin (asthma).

Stress is above all the worst cause of insomnia. By utilizing the techniques above you could decrease stress and say goodbye to insomnia.

Chapter 16: Practical Eft Session For

Overcoming Anxiety

The good news is that you can overcome anxiety.

I have studied a wide range of personal development and self help techniques over the last 15 years. And as a practitioner for a range of techniques such as; neuro linguistic programming, clinical hypnotherapy, thought field therapy and emotional freedom technique – I find EFT to be the simplest self help technique that we can use to overcome and eliminate emotional issues. I use the technique frequently, even on myself, when new situations or challenges come up which cause either uneasiness or nervousness.

Aim to use this technique on both your current emotional issues which are causing you to feel anxious but also to keep the technique handy to use on any future situations which may cause you to feel uneasy or nervous – in order to give you the freedom to live the life that you truly deserve.

Always bear in mind that there may be more than one issue which causes you to feel anxious, as I say, "like peeling an onion" in this case just deal with one emotional issue at a time. It's well worth the effort, and so are you!

The practical session

While focusing on the emotional issue associated with your anxiety;

Before we go through this practical exercise – remember to take full responsibility for your own wellbeing before doing any form of intervention like this.

Rate the level of discomfort

First of all think of the emotional issue i.e. the anxiety - and give it a rating of between 0 and 10. 10 being the highest level of discomfort and 0 being no discomfort at all. Make a note of this number. Don't concern yourself about being exact here, normally your gut feel will be accurate enough, as this is used to determine the reduction in the intensity of the

 discomfort after each tapping exercise.

Follow the exercise below by tapping on the relevant tapping point (4 – 6 taps) and repeating the words in bold - while tapping.

While focussing on the discomfort associated with the anxiety;

1. Tapping on the Karate chop point
Even though I feel anxious – I choose to love, accept and respect myself

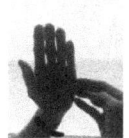

2. Tapping on the Karate chop point
Even though I feel anxious – I choose to love, accept and respect myself.

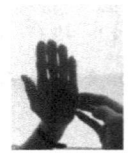

3. Tapping on the Karate chop point
Even though I feel anxious, I feel anxious around others, sometimes I feel anxious all be myself. I'd much rather feel good. And even though I feel so anxious – I choose to deeply and completely love, accept and respect myself and anyone else who may have contributed to my anxiety

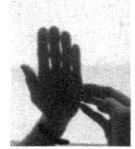

4. Tapping on the beginning of the eyebrow
This anxiety

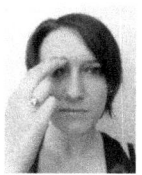

5. Tapping on the side of the eye
This anxiety

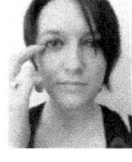

6. Tapping on the under eye point
☐All these anxious feelings

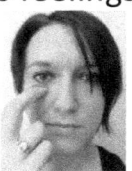

7. Tapping under the nose
☐All this nervousness

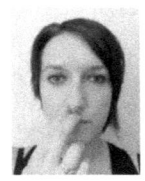

8. Tapping on the chin
☐All these anxious behaviours

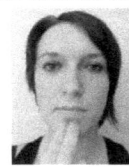

9. Tapping on the collar bone
☐All this anxiety

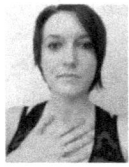

10. Tapping under the arm
☐choose to clear it

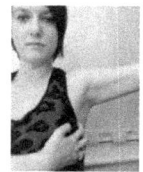

11. Tapping on the top of the head
☐ As much as I can

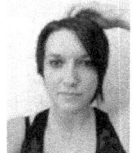

12. Tapping on the beginning of the eyebrow
I choose to let go of this anxiety

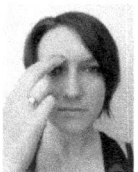

13. Tapping on the side of the eye
I choose to let go of this nervousness

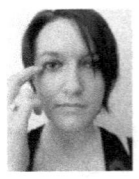

14. Tapping on the under eye point
I choose to let go of all this discomfort

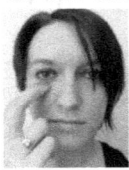

15. Tapping under the nose
I feel so uncomfortable at times

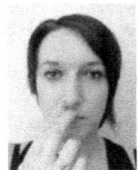

16. Tapping on the chin
I feel so uncomfortable in certain situations

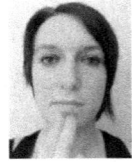

17. Tapping on the collar bone
 I just want to escape

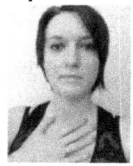

18. Tapping under the arm
It feels like it's just too much for me at times

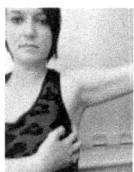

19. Tapping on the top of the head
I just can't stand feeling this way

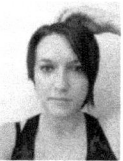

20. Tapping on the beginning of the eyebrow
I am so anxious

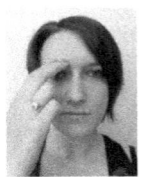

21. Tapping on the side of the eye
I am so uncomfortable

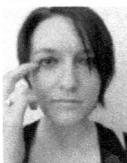

22. Tapping on the under eye point
And I choose to release this feeling

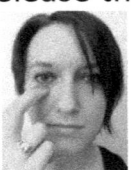

23. Tapping under the nose
I choose to release it at a cellular level

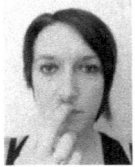

24. Tapping on the chin
I choose to release it all the way back through my past

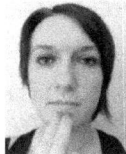

25. Tapping on the collar bone
Back through all of the times when I have been anxious

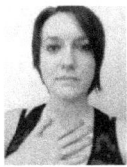

26. Tapping under the arm
All of those times when I just didn't know what to do with myself

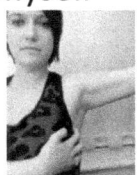

 27. Tapping on the top of the head
And I appreciate that a part of me

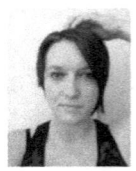

28. Tapping on the beginning of the eyebrow
Is trying to take care of me

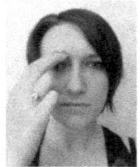

29. Tapping on the side of the eye
By telling me to run away

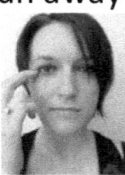

30. Tapping on the under eye point
There's just some part of me

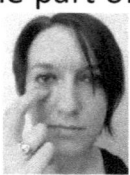

31. Tapping under the nose
That doesn't feel safe

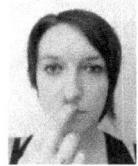

32. Tapping on the chin
A part of me that feels that I am in a fearful situation

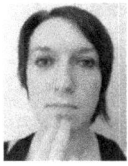

33. Tapping on the collar bone
And I need to escape

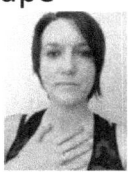

34. Tapping under the arm
So what is it that I am afraid of?

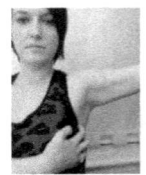

35. Tapping on the top of the head
What am I so afraid of?

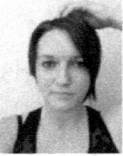

 36. Tapping on the beginning of the eyebrow
Am I afraid of other people or certain situations?

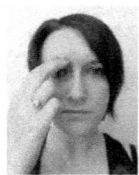

37. Tapping on the side of the eye
Am I afraid of what they'll think of me or what may happen?

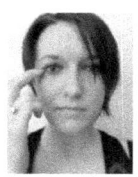

38. Tapping on the under eye
Am I afraid of what others may do or say to me?

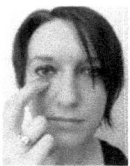

39. Tapping under the nose
What am I basing this fear on?

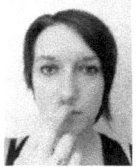

40. Tapping on the chin
And maybe a part of me says

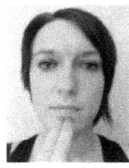

41. Tapping on the collar bone
Oh I've got some very real reasons to base it on

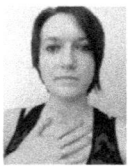

42. Tapping under the arm
⬜ have some real evidence that I'm not safe

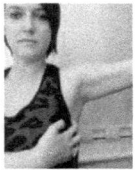

43. Tapping on the top of the head
And I'm choosing to go through that evidence

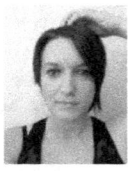

44. Tapping on the beginning of the eyebrow

And clear whatever I can

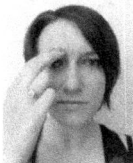

45. Tapping on the side of the eye
☐And that doesn't mean that I'll become silly or stupid

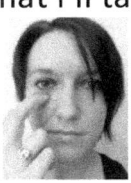

46. Tapping on the under eye
It doesn't mean that I'll take stupid risks

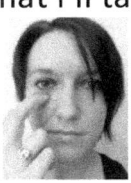

47. Tapping under the nose
I'm just allowing myself

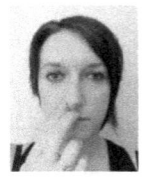

48. Tapping on the chin
☐To clear up any misunderstandings

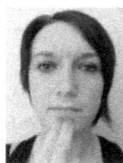

49. Tapping on the collar bone
Because maybe some of these past events

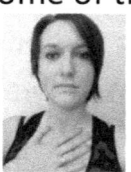

50. Tapping under the arm
☐Were not nearly as fearful as I thought they were

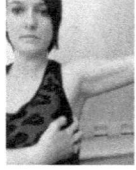

51. Tapping on the top of the head
And maybe they were

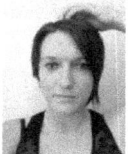

52. Tapping on the beginning of the eyebrow
But I'm not in the same kind of situation any more

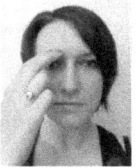

53. Tapping on the side of the eye
Part of me is just making certain

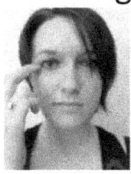

54. Tapping on the under eye
And that's ok

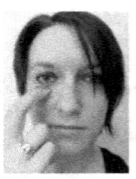

55. Tapping under the nose
I'm not wrong or bad

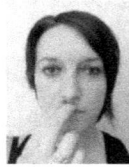

56. Tapping on the chin
I just choose to see

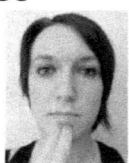

57. Tapping on the collar bone
Whether I'm depriving myself for no good
reason

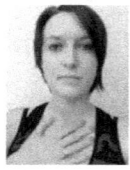

58. Tapping under the arm
After all I don't have to hang out with other people if I don't want to

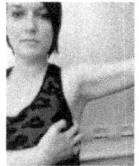

59. Tapping on the top of the head
But maybe I choose to?

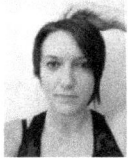

60. Tapping on the beginning of the eyebrow
Maybe I choose to connect with others

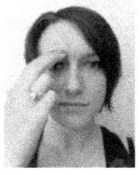

61. Tapping on the side of the eye
So I'm letting go of this anxiety

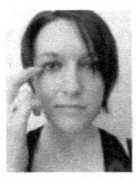

62. Tapping on the under eye
I'm letting go of this fear

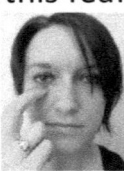

63. Tapping under the nose
I'm letting go of any past embarrassment

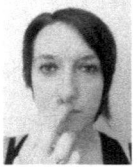

64. Tapping on the chin
I'm letting go of any guilt or shame

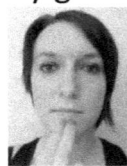

65. Tapping on the collar bone

Letting go of this discomfort

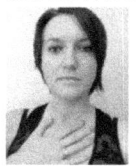

66. Tapping under the arm
I deserve to be here

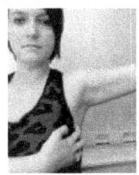

67. Tapping on the top of the head
I have a right to be here

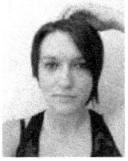

68. Tapping on the beginning of the eyebrow
I choose to believe that I am amazing

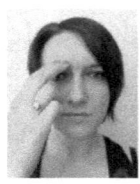

69. Tapping on the side of the eye
I enjoy connecting with others

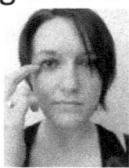

70. Tapping on the under eye
And I choose to feel confident connecting
with others

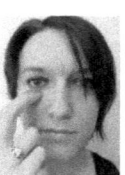

71. Tapping under the nose
I choose to allow myself the freedom to
connect with others

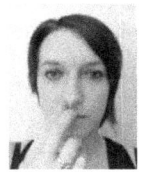

72. Tapping on the chin
I choose to feel safe and at ease

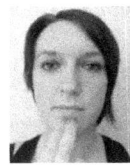

73. Tapping on the collar bone
I choose to feel comfortable and confident

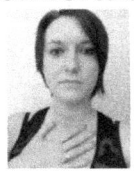

74. Tapping under the arm
I choose to feel calm and confident

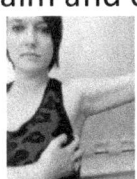

75. Tapping on the top of the head

In my body, mind and spirit

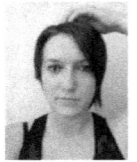

Now take a deep breath... and exhale!
Now once again;
Rate the level of discomfort
Think of the emotional issue i.e. the anxiety - and give it a rating again of between 0 and 10. Has the intensity come down from the first rating? If the rating has reduced (it usually falls by 2 – 3 points – but sometimes more) then repeat the exercise until the rating falls to a rating of 2 or below.
If the rating has not reduced, try the exercise again. If there is still no reduction in the rating, then try changing the initial setup phrase i.e. "Even though I feel very nervous, I choose to love, accept and

respect myself" and then follow the rest of the exercise through.

Or it may be that during the exercise a specific thought has come up for you – in that case, insert that particular thought or phrase into the exercise

For example;

If the thought that came up was "I am afraid of being alone"

At step 36 you could replace the phrase with;

"I am afraid of being alone"

And at step 72 you could replace the phrase with

"I choose to feel safe and at ease when I am alone."

Then repeat the exercise using this phrase and rate the level of intensity afterwards and repeat as necessary, until the rating falls to 2 or below.

Just play around with it and see what works best for you, it can't hurt – it can only help.

Note

It's important to use the ideas, thoughts or phrases which come up for you, as these will be linked to your specific emotional issues.

After the exercise

When you use EFT - you will most likely find, that other issues come forward, either while you are dealing with an issue, or perhaps after an issue is resolved (almost like peeling an onion – layer after layer). When that happens, use EFT to deal with

one emotional issue at a time – until you've peeled the onion, so to speak.

Chapter 17: Giving Positivity

"We make a living by what we get, but we make a life by what we give."
Winston Churchill

In this chapter, we will be discussing the importance of doing good deeds and why you should start doing them to accomplish a happier life.

As you see, many religions and cultures value the act of helping others. Helping others by doing good deeds in life is important as it can make all the difference for someone else and in-turn make you feel good.

Selfless acts, in general, make you feel positive about yourself and spread positivity to others, the more positivity we have in this world the easier it is to be happy. Compassion is one of life's most wonderful feelings and gifts. It will make a big difference in your life and happiness.

145

Why Do Good Deeds?

Doing good deeds are very powerful and there are many benefits from it. Goodness pays you back equally in the future as well as right in the present moment. Spreading positivity to others only gives great outcomes, happiness, and love. These days it is of growing importance to give positive energy more than ever as people, especially in bigger cities, are becoming more self-centered, private and isolated. To change the world, and to help pave your journey to happiness we need to start doing it right now.

Doing good deeds will also come back to you. You should never do something just because you think you will get something back, but it's mostly our human nature. Habitually doing genuine good deeds will bring positivity into your life that you cannot imagine. It almost recreates itself. That friend that you helped out will strengthen the friendship and when you need them most they won't think twice and will offer their own form of genuine good deeds. That elderly lady you helped bring her heavy bags to her car at the supermarket might boost your self-esteem so much that you end up being 10x happier that whole week and that might lead you to talk or meet someone who will help you get a better job in the future. Anything is possible. The point is that when you feel better about yourself (genuine good deeds will give you that) you will start to exude more positive energy into the world in which people around you will respond to. It will strengthen your relationships, your self-esteem, and your attractiveness to others. Do your best to help people with something small as much as possible and notice the results.

Here are some ideas of how you can give positive energy or do some good deeds in this world:
- Donate to charity
- Help a friend in need

- Volunteer for something you're passionate about
- Buy a gift or flowers for your mother or grandmother
- Write a thank-you note to someone who won't expect it
- Compliment others
- Hold the door for others
- Say hello to others and smile
- Pick up trash from the sidewalk
- Help someone who seems to be struggling with something

It is also very easy to get absorbed by our own personal gains and our very own well-being, try not to do good deeds solely for your own happiness but direct your energy to help boost others' happiness. By stepping outside of our daily routines and comfort zones to boost the happiness of others will in-turn boost our own happiness as well. It can also become viral as this is the prime way to spread happiness through the human race. You should try to do one nice thing for someone each day if possible. This might be simple as greeting someone with a nice welcoming smile, helping a coworker with a specific task, lending a pencil to someone in class, or just by calling your parents and tell them how much you love them. Go on and try it and you will replenish yourself with such positivity and happiness in your life.

Chapter 18: Getting Over Depression

To get over depression, you have to do the exact opposite of what we have just discussed in the previous chapter. Remember as a human being, you have the power of choice, the power to choose what you want.

Just like in the first phase, there is a vast amount of information flying around, for ease of understanding we are going to use the same scenario of Sam but only this time we will assume that he is positive in his thoughts.

Conscious mind

The conscious mind, is the thinking mind, So Sam will entertain thoughts based on the information he is exposed to. Just like it was mentioned earlier on, there information we get exposed to is neither good nor bad, it's just is. The deciding factor is how one uses this information.

So Sam might be bullied, other kids might be laughing at him for not having the

latest gadgets and all of the cool stuff. Instead of Sam getting worried about all of this, Sam choses to entertain ideas such as
- Why is he an easy target for bullies?
- Why do some kids have the latest of everything?
- Ways of making money as a student
- How to stand against a bully
- How much does the latest gadgets costs
- What activities can one partake on to make new friends

In short Sam will seek understanding, once you gain understanding of something or a situation, you can be able to manipulate it in your favor.

So Sam can seek understanding from his friends back at home, family members' guidance counselor, pastor or teachers.

Upon seeking understanding, Sam will learn that bullies are just cowards who are just seeking to prove dominance, he will learn that if you stand up to them, they will just shrink, he will learn that they seek vulnerable kids and they go out to them, they never attack groups.

Sam will also learn that people are from different families, some families are wealthy some are not, interestingly he will learn that not all kids who have the latest gadgets get money from their households, some of them work during holidays, they deliver newspapers, they seek means of making money in their community.

Most importantly Sam will learn that the reason he is finding it difficult to make friends is because he is not a member of any social circle. when he thinks these thoughts frequently, they will be impressed upon his subconscious mind.

Subconscious mind

Since these thoughts are positive and inspiring in nature, they will be impressed as faith not fear upon the subconscious mind. The funny thing about both faith and fear is the fact that they require you to believe in something you do not see.

So Sam will start to believe that if he can stand up to his bullies they will stop harassing him, if he finds a small circle of friends, no bully can attack him. He also believes that if he can find a job during holidays, he can make enough money to buy all the gadgets he wants. Faith based on understanding is the key to freedom.

The faith will be expressed in the body as well-being, not as anxiety.

Well-being is expressed not suppressed. So Sam will act based on his belief (faith), he will defend himself and stand up against his bullies, he will decide to join a team, either the swimming, football or volley ball team. He might be horrible at playing the sport, but he will make friends and in no time he will belong somewhere.

He will seek ways to make money during holidays. He will deliver newspapers, work in local grocery stores, and when he goes back to school, he will have some pocket money he can use to buy what he wants.

When you achieve what you believe in, you will be at ease, calm and happy. You will be creative and you will be able to create more situations that will favor you. You will be the master of your fate and the captain of your destiny, no adverse condition will scare you because you will now be aware that the power to create rests completely with you.

Chapter 19: How To Meditate?

Choose the right place and time.

The first step is to find an appropriate place for you to practice. It does not have to be a garden that is full of chirping birds, though it is best done close to nature. I prefer to go to the beach and find a quiet spot where no one else is around, so I can hear the waves in the background, it really helps calm me during meditation. Or, a quiet spot in your house can very well do. Some people would prefer soothing music in the background and some would just prefer the quiet. Proper clothing should also be worn during meditation. Tight fit clothes would only keep the body tight and contracted, it is therefore suggested that comfortable clothes that are fitting just right should be used during meditation. Most importantly, choose a setting that could work for you.

Meditation is best practiced before the start and end of the day. If your schedule permits, it would be recommended that meditation is done during the morning after waking up and during the night, before going to sleep. The mediation practice would help clear the mind and start the day with the right perspective. During the night, it would help release all the tensions you have built up that were experienced during the whole day, letting you feel renewed and cleansed for the next morning.

The meditation length is not particular. If you have more time to spare, then you can meditate longer, if it is a busy day ahead, then you can make it shorter. The important thing is that you know your goal for the meditation and focus on that goal. Breathe.

There are times when you would not find it easy to concentrate and just be lost in your thoughts, this situation is normal. Just go back to your breathing and try to focus on that, you can try to focus on a mantra if you need to. Listen to your breathing and feel every part of your body as you inhale and exhale. This way, you are focusing on your body more and not on other thoughts.

Commit.

Regular practice of meditation is best suggested to fully acquire its benefits. It will help if you assign a specific time and decide before hand how long you should practice. You can choose to meditate early in the morning and if you can, before going to sleep again. It does not have to be a full hour, a 15-minute meditation practice every day can be of benefit already. The important thing is that you take time during your day to just close your eyes and be free from all the thoughts that you have.

Chapter 20: Yoga Poses For Depression

STANDING FORWARD BEND

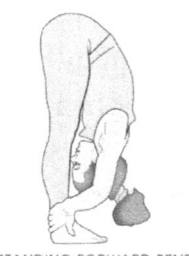

STANDING FORWARD BEND

Procedure:

Stand straight with your spine erect and your hands on the hips.

Inhale as you slowly raise your hands above your head. Let the palms face each other.

With exhalation, bend at your hips to bring your body down.

Slowly bring your hands towards the ground and place your palms near your feet. Do not bend your knees.

Try to bend as much as possible so that your spine stretches well to make a perfect forward bend.

Do not rest your forehead on your knees. You need to leave your head hanging down towards the floor.

While returning to position, bring your hands to your hips and then rise with an inhalation.

Benefits:

This pose helps calm the brain.

It relieves fatigue, stress and depression.

Abdominal organs are stimulated which improves digestion.

The functioning of liver and kidneys are enhanced.

It addresses problems related to menopause.

Note: Those suffering from back injury need to be cautious while practicing this asana.

INVERTED LEG POSE

The pose is also known as LEGS-UP-THE-WALL POSE. The pose derived this name from the fact that some people use wall to support their legs in doing the pose.

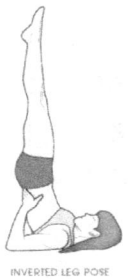

INVERTED LEG POSE

Procedure:

Lie down with your legs stretched and hands by your sides.

Lift your legs straight up to an angle of 90 degrees.

Let the feet be straight so that the soles face upward.

Raise your pelvis slightly and with your hands to support, maintain a 45-degree posture of your waist from your shoulders.

Ensure that you do not go straight as in Shoulder Stand.

Remain in the pose for a while before returning to position.

160

If the practitioner finds it difficult to achieve the pose with the support of hands, use of pillows or folded blankets are suggested. The supporting block can be placed under the pelvis to give a rise.

Duration: You can remain in the pose for 3 minutes. However, you need to consider your medical condition as you determine the duration of the pose.

Benefits:

It improves blood flow in the head area. This helps in relieving depression and anxiety. It is good for migraine and headaches caused by poor oxygenation and blood flow.

It stimulates the nervous system, helping you become physically and mentally fit. Youthfulness and vigor can be maintained by practicing the pose regularly.

Abdominal organs receive excellent toning and stimulation. This helps in curing digestive disorders including constipation.

It is a great alternative cure for insomnia. Those who suffer from sleeplessness are sure to find remedy in this pose.

This is an excellent pose for women as it cures menstrual cramps and helps in addressing problems related to menopause.

It helps in treating swollen ankles and varicose vein problems.

Note: Those who suffer from back or neck injury should not do the pose without support. Those with severe eye problems need to consult their physician first before proceeding with the pose.

UPWARD FACING DOG POSE

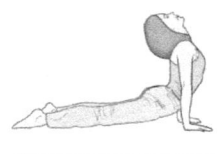

UPWARD FACING DOG POSE

Procedure:

Lie down on your stomach. Stretch your legs, have the top of your feet on the mat and let the hands be by the sides.

Place your palms near either side of your waist and space out your fingers. Now, you will note that your forearms are perpendicular to the ground.

With inhalation, press your palms on the floor as you straighten your hands and lift your body and head.

Your palms and your feet will be supporting your body and your thighs and knees should be a few inches above the mat. Your wrists should be in line with your shoulders.

Press your tailbone towards the pubis. Lift the pubis towards your navel.

Let the shoulders be drawn back. Let your neck be aligned to your spine.

Exhale as you lower your body to the mat.

Duration: 15 to 30 seconds

Benefits:

This pose is helpful in treating mild depression and fatigue.

It relieves stress and depression associated with menopause.

The pose strengthens the arms and wrists.

It addresses asthmatic complaints.

It improves the functioning of the abdominal organs.

Note:

Those with severe back injury should not practice this pose.

Those who are suffering from carpal tunnel syndrome should refrain from practicing this pose.

Do not practice this pose if you have a headache.

DOWNWARD FACING DOG POSE

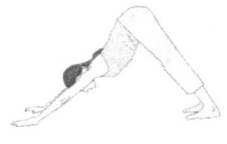

DOWNWARD FACING DOG POSE

Procedure:

Go on fours on the floor with your knees and palms on the floor.

Your wrists should be in line with your shoulders and your knees with your hips.

Lift your knees and let your feet touch the ground firmly.

Raise your hips. Now you would resemble an inverted "V" shape.

Do not bend your knees and elbows.

Return to position.

Duration: 15 to 30 seconds

Benefits:

This pose works wonders for mental depression; it calms the mind.

Your spine is stretched and stress is relieved.

The pose strengthens arms and legs.

WARRIOR POSE

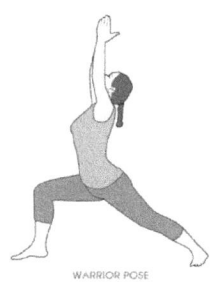

WARRIOR POSE

Procedure:

Stand straight with legs apart maintaining a distance of about four feet.

Keep your left foot at 90-degree angle towards left side. Turn your right foot 45 degrees towards left side.

Turn the upper part of your body towards left without changing the position of your legs.

Bend the left knee to bring it in straight line above the left foot.

Stretch your arms sideways and slowly raise them and keep your palms together.

Ensure that your hands are stretched well enough so that you feel the pull in your shoulders and waist.

Bend your neck backwards and look at the closed palms.

Slowly return to position.

Duration: 30 seconds to 1 minute

Benefits:

It relaxes the mind and improves concentration.

It is a great pose for legs and joints. It works on thighs, calf muscles, ankles, shoulders and neck and strengthens them.

It tones the back muscles.

The pose improves balance and lung functions.

It is a good pose for people with sciatic problems.

Note: Those with heart conditions and high blood pressure should refrain from performing this asana. Those with neck problems don't need to bend backwards. Instead, they can keep their head straight and gaze forward.

COW POSE AND CAT POSE

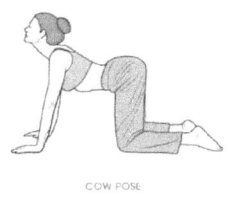

COW POSE

167

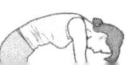

Procedure:

Cow and Cat Pose form a perfect combination as they blend excellently well to produce amazing results.

Kneel down on the floor.

Place your arms in front of you and lift your body. Keep the back straight to resemble a table.

Knees should be straight below the hips.

The wrists should fall in line with shoulders.

Inhale deeply and raise your sit bones and chest high toward the ceiling. The abdomen should slowly expand and go towards the ground.

Lift your head and look straight ahead. This is the **Cow Pose**.

Now, slowly exhale and round your back effectively in opposite direction.

Fix your gaze on your belly. Expel all air from the lungs by bringing the belly button up towards your spine. This is the **Cat Pose**.

Duration: 20 seconds (3 times)

Benefits:

It helps stabilize emotions; it calms the mind.

The pose stretches the neck and strengthens it.

Relieves stress in the neck and shoulder.

It improves digestion.

Note: Those with knee and neck injury should be extra cautious while practicing this pose.

COBRA POSE

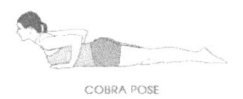
COBRA POSE

Procedure:

Lie on your stomach, face downwards. Keep your palms by the sides near your chest bending at the elbows.

Inhale, lift your head, chest and back up to waist.

Your hands should be perpendicular to the ground.

Keep your head straight, pull back your shoulders thus expanding your chest.

Return to position.

Duration: 20 seconds (2 times)

Benefits:

Helpful for people suffering from mild depression.

It relieves fatigue in women during menstrual cycle.

Flexibility of the lower back improves.

Upper back muscles are toned.

Relieves neck and shoulder pain.

Digestion is improved.

Note:

Those with back injury should refrain from practicing this pose.

People suffering from carpal tunnel syndrome should not practice this asana.
LOCUST POSE

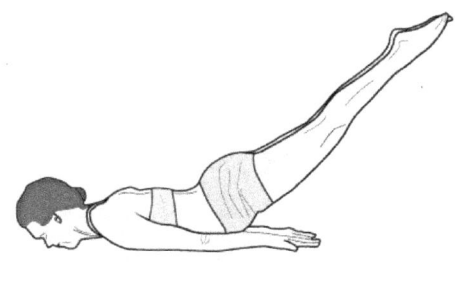

LOCUST POSE

Procedure:

Lie on your stomach with your chin on the ground and hands on the sides.

Let the palm face down.

Inhale, lift both your legs upward as high as possible without bending your knees.

Exhale and return to position.

Duration: 20 seconds (2 times)

Benefits:

The asana rejuvenates your body and helps in relieving depression.

It tones the lower half of the body.

The asana tones the lumbo-sacral bones-good for lower back problems.

It also helps in treating upper back problems.

As abdominal organs are toned, the functioning of kidneys, liver and pancreas is enhanced.

It is great for sciatica and slip disc problems.

This posture helps in treating varicose vein problems.

THE BOW POSE

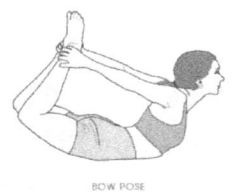

BOW POSE

Procedure:

Lie on your stomach.

Bend your legs at the knees, raise your thighs and hold the ankles with your hands.

Your body now rests on your abdomen and your spine is arched.

Return to position by releasing the ankles and placing your legs and hands down.

Duration: 15 seconds (2 times)

Benefits:

It helps in reducing anxiety by toning the Solar Plexus Chakra.

Excess fat in the abdomen is removed.

It cures constipation and intestinal disorders; it improves digestion.

Improves the flexibility of the spine.

It is an excellent posture for the middle back.

Shoulders and neck are stretched; upper back is relaxed.

Good for upper back pain caused by breathing disorders.

It is a good pose for the diabetic.

Note:

Those with severe back problems should seek the guidance of yoga professional before performing this posture.

Though this asana offers great relief from various stomach and back problems, people suffering from such conditions should practice this posture strictly under supervision.

SEATED FORWARD BEND POSTURE

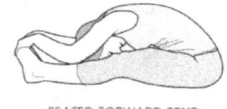

SEATED FORWARD BEND

Procedure:

Sit with the legs outstretched and spine erect.

Inhale as you raise your arms.

Exhale and bend forward to touch your toes.

Place your head on the knees.

Do not bend your knees.

Duration: 20 counts (3 times)

Benefits:

The posture relaxes the mind and helps in relieving mild depression and stress.

Extra inches around the waist are shed. Belly fat is reduced.

This posture is effective for both upper and lower back pain as the spinal nerves are toned and blood circulation improves in the back.

Vertebral column alignment improves with practice.

It strengthens the spine and back muscles.

Entire body is relaxed as the muscles from neck to feet are stretched.

Note:

Those with severe back ailments should refrain from practicing this posture.

People with slipped disc problems should also avoid practicing this asana.

Though it is good for liver, if a person has enlarged liver, he has to avoid doing this posture.

BRIDGE POSE

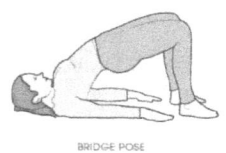

BRIDGE POSE

Procedure:

Lie on your back.
Place your arms by your sides with palms facing down.
Bending your knees, place your feet on the ground. Maintain hip width between your feet.
Keeping the hands on the ground, raise your hips as high as possible.
Retain this pose for a while and return to position.
Duration: 10 seconds (3 times)
Benefits:

It helps in treating depression.
It relaxes the shoulders.
It helps in relieving fatigue and neck pain.
The pose strengthens the spine and back.
Helpful for people with breathing disorders.
CAMEL POSE

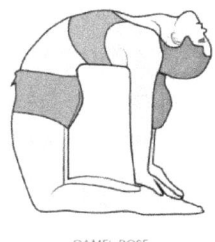

CAMEL POSE

Procedure:
Sit in Vajrasana posture, that is, you need to form a 'V' shape by spacing out your heels and the big toes touching each other.
Raise your hands above your head and bend backwards as you inhale.
Hold your ankles with your hands as you exhale. Your spine should arch well.
Return to the position.

Duration: 30 seconds (2 times)

Benefits:

The pose is good for anxiety and stress.

Concentration and memory improves due to a better blood flow in the brain.

It is good for upper back pain; it relieves stress in the neck and upper back.

The posture is good for insomnia, backache and neck pain.

Pulling the shoulders backwards while performing this posture helps to relax the shoulders and provides good massage for the upper back.

As the lung performance improves, breathing disorders are cured and this helps in relieving upper back pain caused by breathing disorders.

Chest and abdomen are stretched; the abdominal organs are massaged.

Note:

Those with severe and chronic back conditions should avoid this asana.

Those with migraine, high and low blood pressure should not attempt doing this posture.

HALF-SPINAL TWIST

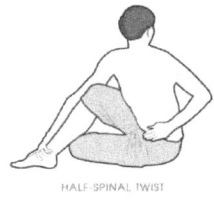

HALF-SPINAL TWIST

Procedure:

Bend your left leg, bring it over the right knee and place your left foot beside your right knee on the ground.

Fold your right leg and bring the heel closer to your left buttock. Keep the right leg to the ground in resting position.

Raise your right hand over the left leg and grasp the big toe of your left foot.

Inhale, slowly twist your trunk as you exhale and gaze over your left shoulder.

Bring your left hand around your waist.
Keep the palm facing outside.

Return to position.

Repeat with the alternate hand and leg.

Duration: 30 seconds (2 times)

Benefits:

The pose helps in detoxifying the body and in relieving depression.

It helps treat nervous disorders.

The posture prevents urinary tract disorders.

The functioning of spinal cord is improved.

Pelvic region is greatly benefited by this asana as blood circulation improves and sufficient supply of oxygen and nutrients is guaranteed.

The pose improves the flexibility of spine as it is twisted from base to the neck- good for upper back and lower back pain

The back muscles are stretched and hips become supple.

Note: Those suffering from spinal cord problems should be cautious in practicing this posture.

CHILD POSE

Procedure:

Kneel on the ground and sit on your heels.

Bring your trunk forward and place your forehead on the ground.

Place your hands by your sides to reach your ankle.

Alternately, you can stretch your hands in front of you on the floor.

Return to position.

Duration: 20 – 30 seconds (2 times)

Benefits:

It relaxes your body and mind.

The pose strengthens the spine.

It is good for the entire back as the pose gives a complete stretch.

It stretches your back, hips and thighs and relaxes the spine and shoulders.

The stretch helps to relax the neck when the forehead is rested on the floor. The pose helps in treating neck pain.

Note:

Those with knee injury and ankle problems should avoid practicing this pose.
People with high blood pressure and heart ailments should avoid this pose.

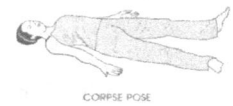

CORPSE POSE

CORPSE POSE

Procedure:

Lie on your back with your feet slightly apart.
Place your hands at the sides but a bit away from your body.
Keep your eyes closed and let your body be completely relaxed.
Inhale and exhale slowly.
Duration: When this posture is done at the end of the yoga session of around 30

minutes duration, you need to relax for at least 10 minutes.

Benefits:

This posture offers complete relaxation for the body and mind, thus, stress is relieved.

Muscles are relaxed.

Body and mind are rejuvenated.

Brain function is improved.

It helps in relieving neck pain caused by fatigue.

It helps in treating insomnia.

Chapter 21: Implementing Necessary Lifestyle Modifications

Addressing your triggers means that you need to cultivate specific and concrete measures designed to rid yourself of anxiety. These measures are all part of the necessary lifestyle modifications that you need to implement in order to reclaim your life back and improve your overall physical, emotional and mental well-being. Begin by dealing with stress. Here are ways to make sure you will not get weighed down again by stress in the future:

1) Develop effective time management techniques such as building a schedule and adhering to deadlines.

2) Prioritize your tasks and organize them according to hierarchy.

3) Set reasonable and realistic expectations for yourself.

4) Do away with perfectionism

5) Learn to say no. Avoid high-stress situations by working within what you are capable of. Otherwise you only set yourself up for failure and disappointment.

6) Learn to relax.

7) Create positive distractions.

To deal with your finances, here are a couple of helpful strategies:

1) Live within your means.

2) Create a budget.

3) Seek the help of a financial counselor if you need to.

4) To improve your overall physical well-being, observe the following:

5) Exercise.

6) Be mindful of your diet. In this regard, avoid caffeinated food items.

7) Learn easy relaxation methods such as deep breathing, meditation, yoga, or Tai'Chi.

8) Sleep well.

Another great way to overcome your anxieties is by creating a strong support group. On this end, remember to build healthy and dynamic relationships with your family, friends and the people around you. As mentioned in the previous chapters, dysfunctional relationships from both your past and present can trigger anxiety-filled responses from you.

It is therefore important that you build a strong sense of connection and stable channels of communication with them. This will not only minimize your tendencies to harbor a sense of mistrust toward them, it will also allow you to foster greater peace of mind.

Most importantly, learn to face your fears. The entire concept of anxiety is anchored on the idea of "avoidance," where you choose to build an impregnable wall between you and everything else as a way of avoiding the need to confront whatever it is that you are running away from.

But dodging your issues does not in any way address any of your concerns. Rather, this tendency to escape through anxiety-filled responses only aggravates the situation for you and the people around you.

Chapter 22: Becoming A Socially Connected Introvert – With Ease

I read the introverts forums, I watch the comments, and I feel a little dismayed. "Why won't people leave me alone?" "I don't like small talk, so I avoid people." "Being around people is just so exhausting that I spend all my free time alone." "I hate even the thought of networking."

One gets the impression that all introverts are grumpy, asocial and even hostile to people who desire more stimulation and activity in their lives (OK, extroverts). Unfortunately, good health and success are tied to the high quality of the relationships we form. Isolation is not. It doesn't have to be that hard. Fortunately, I know introverts who are highly successful in personal and professional life, especially relationships.

A story was told of a famous woman who is an introvert who has a wealth of supportive friends and a successful professional life. Everywhere she goes, she seems to encounter someone who knows and likes her. If they don't know her already, they will soon like her. An outgoing extrovert? No, a lifelong introvert, who values her private time, makes it clear to others that she does so, and withdraws and uses meditation frequently to clarify life's problems.

The lessons she models are important ones, because the people who "just want to be left alone" may be nonplussed to discover that they nevertheless need support, such as a drive home from a hospital after a procedure, a place to stay when their home has become temporarily uninhabitable, support for a bright idea, or even just a hug. And if you have a dream or a vision: nobody gets there alone. We all need support, and to get support you need to connect.

How she does it is a model for introverts everywhere. Here are some key guidelines:

Look for similarities, not differences.

It's too easy to see someone else as abrasive or exhausting. Try to look for something you have in common with another person, or at least something likeable - perhaps a characteristic you'd like to have, such as a way of making people smile, or putting them at their ease.

Thoughtfulness: your Secret Weapon

Thinking deeply and noticing subtleties are real introvert skills. Too often we misuse them; our deep thinking becomes rumination, in which we obsess over and over about our inadequacies or embarrassments. The subtleties we may latch on to are other people's negative reactions to things we do or say, rather than insights about the other people. What about changing that to look outward and see other people for who they really are, then think of how you can connect?

Reaching out and sharing doesn't have to be exhausting.

You don't have to sign up for big, noisy events, such as following the crowd to happy hour, to be socially connected.

Invite a colleague or neighbor to have coffee or tea: a one-on-one encounter in which you can find out more about the other person. You can take charge of the time, length and setting of the event.

Connecting doesn't even have to take that much activity, nor do you even have to be physically present. It can only take a minute or so, sometimes even a second, to send thoughtful notes that are easy and quick. Keep some great stationery or cards on hand, then comment on birthdays, anniversaries, and especially successes.

Too busy to find cards and notepaper? Send one of those animated online cards, but make sure you add a personal note.

Set up a calendar which sends you reminders of other people's special events: birthdays, anniversaries.

Special hint to make you special to others: take some time to make the message personal - for example, not just "congratulations," but something like "I knew your ability to focus and be dedicated would pay off like this."

Her way is to keep a list of people she knows and their tastes. During this recent trip, in April, she carried her Christmas list for next year, filling her suitcase with colorful bookmarks, soaps, and trinkets with which to delight her relatives, friends, neighbors, colleagues. All year long she picks up things that she thinks will delight people on that list. Most items are neither large nor expensive, but they are truly insightful. Her choices are very apt!

Having human contacts and arranging that those contacts don't drain you of energy can keep you healthier and happier in so many ways.

Here are some of the consequences of the good social network she has set up:

☐ She loves to travel, and has a host of friends to mind the cat and water the plants when she is away.

☐ She also has a number of friends in other countries with whom she can connect when she next visits.

☐ When she needs something, whether it is a new printer or a new sink, someone in her network seems to know exactly where to get it.

☐ And recently, she started a new small business. With no advertising, not even a website, she had two clients in the first week. Some entrepreneurs agonize over how to attain visibility. She just does it naturally - one contact at a time.

So can you.

Chapter 23: What Is Stress?

According to the American Institute of Stress, 1 out of 5 Americans experience "extreme stress." 60% of all human disease and illnesses are due to stress, particularly stroke, heart disease, and heart attacks. 44% of people who are stressed also experience corresponding sleep loss. 75% of doctors' visits are for stress-triggered symptoms.

Stress can be defined as "the body's response to changes that create taxing demands." A stressor is defined as the internal and/or environmental cause that triggers the body's response. According to health professionals, stress can be either a positive or negative experience. Healthy stress is referred to as "eustress," while harmful stress is referred to as "distress." Although each individual responds differently to a given stressor, there are certain general stressors that individuals categorize as either "positive stressors" or "negative stressors."

Positive Personal Stressors:

Buying a house

Moving

Going on Vacation

New job

Learning a new hobby

Holidays

Taking classes

Relationship changes (i.e. marriage)

A work promotion or bonus

Having a kid

Retiring

Negative Personal Stressors:

Relational conflicts

Divorce

Loss of a spouse

Break-ups

Loss of contact with friends and/or family

A family death

Legal problems

Financial problems

Sickness or injury
Unemployment
Insomnia or other sleep disorders
Kids having trouble at school
Hospitalization
Emotional or physical abuse
If you are employed, you might experience
some additional negative stressors.
Work-related Negative Stressors:
Commuting
Business Trips
Giving presentations to clients or
coworkers
Ineffective or long business meetings
Job insecurity
Inadequate training to complete daily
tasks
Conflicts with coworkers
From these lists, it is obvious that the
stress you experience is impacted by both
external and internal forces. External
stressors are often circumstances or
something in your environment that

trigger a stress response in your body, such as relationships, work, and home. External forces that can generate stress can also include expectations, responsibilities, and challenges that you experience in a given day. Some internal forces that determine what type of stress you experience (positive or negative) are the amount of sleep you get, your physical health and fitness, and your emotional and mental health. Other internal sources of negative stress can include: worrying about the future, having negative thought patterns, having unrealistic expectations (of self or others), and having personal phobias (fear of heights, death, public speaking, talking with strangers, etc.). Health professionals also cite some personal habits that could contribute to stress, as follows: lack of being assertive, procrastinating, failure to plan ahead, and overscheduling.

Conclusion

Curing your anxiety and panic attacks once and for all is a desired effect for all who suffer with the problem. Before we look at a few tips you must know this one important fact. There is no miracle drug...no pills or any medication that will stop anxiety attacks forever. You, and you alone, will have to be the solution or cure for your own anxiety.

Anxiety attacks, also known as panic attacks, are cause by increased amounts of adrenaline releasing into your bloodstream. A message of fear, real or perceived, is sent to your adrenal gland signaling an emergency situation.

When extreme amounts of adrenaline are released into your body the physical symptoms are such that they can be misinterpreted as a heart attack. Rapid heartbeat, excessive perspiration, pain in the chest and a complete unawareness of what is actually going on around you are all symptoms of a panic attack. It is easy to see how they can be mistaken for symptoms of a heart attack.

Once you have experienced a panic attack the mere thought of having another one can trigger your adrenaline gland into action. Learning to control these fears will help control the frequency of your attacks. But, how is this done?

First, you must learn to relax. I know this is easier said than done. You must convince yourself that panic attacks are from a perceived threat. Nothing bad is really going to happen. Slow, deep breathing will help you relax.

Since most panic attacks are from a feeling of fear you must learn to accept your feelings. Try to rationalize exactly what it is you fear. When you fully understand your fears you can decide whether there is a need for any fear at all.

If you decide your fear is from a real danger, by all means take appropriate action. But, if your fear is not real, only perceived, then you must take measures to eliminate the perception of fear.

Finally, you must eliminate negative thinking. No good can come from constantly worrying about bills or money or family. Stop thinking you are going to have another panic attack, too. Many people say they have had an anxiety attack simple because they thought one was about to occur!

Curing your anxiety and panic attacks will not happen overnight. But, with a little patience you will be able to stop anxiety attacks forever.

CPSIA information can be obtained
at www.ICGtesting.com
Printed in the USA
BVHW051506240720
584534BV00009B/335